The Ophthalmic Surgical Assistant

The Ophthalmic Surgical Assistant

Regina Boess-Lott, RN, CRNO
Administrative Director of Clinical and Laser Services
Total Eye Care Center
Levittown, PA

Sharon Stecik
Practice Administrator
Total Eye Care Center
Levittown, PA

|||| The Basic Bookshelf for Eyecare Professionals

Series Editors: Janice K. Ledford, COMT • Ken Daniels, OD • Robert Campbell, MD

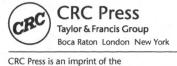

CRC Press
Taylor & Francis Group
Boca Raton London New York

CRC Press is an imprint of the
Taylor & Francis Group, an **informa** business

First published 1999 by SLACK Incorporated

Published 2024 by CRC Press
2385 NW Executive Center Drive, Suite 320, Boca Raton FL 33431

and by CRC Press
4 Park Square, Milton Park, Abingdon, Oxon, OX14 4RN

CRC Press is an imprint of Taylor & Francis Group, LLC

Library of Congress Cataloging-in-Publication Data
Boess-Lott, Regina
   The ophthalmic surgical assistant/ Regina Boess-Lott, Sharon Stecik.
      p. cm. -- (The basic bookshelf for eyecare professionals)
   Includes bibliographical references and index.
   ISBN 1-55642-403-5
   1. Opthalmic assistants. 2. Eye-- Surgery. I. Stecik, Sharon. II. Title. III. Series.
   {DNLM: 1. Eye Diseases--surgery. 2. Ophthalmologic Surgical Procedures-- methods. 3. Ophthalmic Assistants. WW 168 L884o 1999}
   RE72.5.L68 1999
   617.7'1-- dc21
   DNLM/DLC   98-45257

ISBN: 9781556424038 (pbk)
ISBN: 9781003525417 (ebk)

DOI: 10.1201/9781003525417

Dedication

This book is lovingly dedicated to our children,
Robby & Danny
and
Maria & Diane.
They are our inspirations.

Contents

Acknowledgments

There have been many people who have worked with us in the development of this book. Their expertise, advice, guidance, and support have contributed to its completion. Specifically, we would like to thank Jan Ledford, our editor, who has continually encouraged us and kept our focus. The staff and physicians of Total Eye Care Centers who allowed us the flexibility to work on this project, observe them in surgery, and shared their time and expertise, in particular: Barry M. Concool, MD, Judith B. Lavrich, MD, Arunan Sivalingam, MD, Harmon C. Stein, MD, and Mary Siegman, COA. Additionally, Bruce C. Altman, MD, Marc S. Cohen, MD, Sadeer B. Hannush, MD, and Nancy G. Swartz, MD.

We also extend a word of thanks to the OR and nursing staff at Wills Eye Hospital in Philadelphia, Saint Mary Medical Center in Langhorne, PA, and Capital Health Systems at Mercer in Trenton, NJ; specifically Sheila McGuire, RN, Jeanne Hess, RN, Linda Levacs, RN, Dennis Kosar, Pat Kearney, RN, Roberta Samel, RN, and Kathy Prugh, RN. Not to be forgotten, Rose C. Williams, CEBT, Quality Assurance Coordinator of the Lions Eye Bank of Delaware Valley in Philadelphia, and Betsy Osterhout RN, TLC The Laser Center in Mount Laurel, NJ. To everyone who has contributed in any way, we thank you.

About the Authors

Regina Boess-Lott, RN, CRNO

Regina Boess-Lott received her associates degree in nursing science in 1986 from Bucks County Community College in Newtown, PA. In 1991, she achieved the status of a Certified Registered Nurse in Ophthalmology (CRNO). Regina is a member of the American Society of Ophthalmic Registered Nurses (ASORN) and is the current Administrative Director of Clinical and Laser Services for Total Eye Care Centers, based in Levittown, PA. She has over 16 years of experience in the field of ophthalmology, including comprehensive operating room and clinical care.

Sharon Stecik

Sharon Stecik, also a graduate of Bucks County Community College, has been in the field of ophthalmology since 1976. Since 1990, she has held her current position as Practice Administrator at Total Eye Care Centers. A 1983 graduate of the Ophthalmic Technician's Program at the Eye Institute of New Jersey, University of Medicine and Dentistry in Newark, NJ, Sharon has had the opportunity to work in both clinical and surgical care. She is an active member of the American Society of Ophthalmic Administrators.

Introduction

The ophthalmic surgical assistant, referred to as OA throughout this book, has an indispensable role in the surgical suite, whether it is hospital- or office-based. With today's demanding surgical caseload, the need for educated and well-trained technical assistance is of great value to the ophthalmic surgeon. The ultimate success of any surgical procedure is dependent on efficiently orchestrated teamwork (surgeon and personnel) in the operating room (OR) environment. Surgical assisting is ideal for highly motivated individuals with a sense of organization and attention to detail. With the constant development of ophthalmic procedures and instrumentation, it is the responsibility of the surgeon and support personnel to keep abreast of current techniques.

As an important member of the surgical team, ophthalmic surgical assistants contribute to the rewarding process of restoring vision. It is the hope of the authors of this book that those who have chosen this exciting and challenging profession will benefit from this basic reference information we have assembled.

Remember to keep in mind that each ophthalmic surgeon, hospital, and surgical facility follows individual policies and procedures. It is the responsibility of the OA to identify individual protocol and surgeon preferences in all of the ophthalmic sub-specialties. With this text, we have attempted to compile basic guidelines and typical scenarios in ophthalmology.

The Study Icons

The Basic Bookshelf for Eyecare Professionals Series is quality educational material designed for professionals in all branches of eyecare. Because so many of you want to expand your careers, we have made a special effort to include information needed for certification exams. When these study icons appear in the margin of a *Series* book, it is your cue that the material next to the icon (which may be a paragraph or an entire section) is listed as a criteria item for a certification examination. Please use this key to identify the appropriate icon:

OptA	optometric assistant
OptT	optometric technician
OphA	ophthalmic assistant
OphT	ophthalmic technician
OphMT	ophthalmic medical technologist
LV	low vision subspecialty
Srg	ophthalmic surgical assisting subspecialty*
CL	contact lens registry
Optn	opticianry
RA	retinal angiographer

Note: Because this icon applies to the entire book, it will not appear anywhere on the pages.

Chapter 1

Preoperative Counseling and Informed Consent

- Proper patient education is an asset in preoperative and post-operative compliance.

- Informed consent procedures have a medicolegal impact on the ophthalmic surgical candidate.

- The typical informed consent consists of an explanation of the procedure, anesthesia, risks, and complications.

Patient Education: An Essential Tool

An educated patient can be a valuable asset to the ophthalmologist, as knowledge enhances any experience in the ophthalmology practice of today. Informed patients are better prepared to understand their condition and are more compliant during their course of treatment.

There are a variety of instructional modalities available to achieve these goals in the form of printed materials (brochures, posters), audio- or videotapes, anatomical models, and support groups (Figure 1-1). It is advantageous for the surgical counselor to have these materials available during the explanation of surgical procedures, as a patient can relate to a tangible object in conjunction with a verbal explanation. As the surgical patient is often apprehensive about the upcoming procedure, often you will find he or she will retain very little verbal explanation. Therefore, it is also advisable to have a family member present.

Informed Consent

In the litigious environment medicine faces today, it is extremely important that informed consent issues are not treated lightly. Patient consent is an essential and important step in the preoperative process. In addition, explaining the procedures and possible complications gives the physician and assistant another opportunity to establish an open communication process. Allowing ample time for explanation and questions can circumvent any future misunderstandings. Ongoing communication between the physician, staff, and patient further adds to surgical success.

A typical informed consent should consist of a verbal explanation of the procedure, eye involved, anesthesia, risks, and complications. This is documented in the patient chart as well as in a written informed consent. There are many sample documents available through ophthalmological organizations and private companies that can be customized to a particular ophthalmic practice.

Informed consent is a critical step in the process of scheduling the ophthalmic surgical patient. Establishing open patient rapport and meticulous attention to documentation is essential both medicolegally and in the managed care environment governed by the National Committee on Quality Assurance (NCQA) standards of today. Further information can be found in the Basic Bookshelf Series title *Overview of Ocular Surgery and Surgical Counseling*.

Intraoperative Communication

It is not taboo for the patient to speak with the surgeon during the surgical procedure. Appropriate communication techniques need to be explained to the surgical candidate to avoid potential intraoperative disasters. The need to scratch a nose, cough, sneeze, lack of air, or the feeling of claustrophobia under the drape are all common scenarios that can be attended to easily by either the ophthalmic surgical assistant (OA) or the surgeon. If ignored, patient anxiety levels will heighten needlessly. Therefore, careful explanation of what the patient may see, hear, and smell contributes to the ultimate success of the surgical procedure.

Of course, patient privacy must be preserved at all costs. Whatever happens in the OR stays

What the Patient Needs to Know*

OptA

OphA

- You have the right to considerate and special care.

- You have the right to obtain from your physician complete and current information concerning your diagnosis, treatment, and prognosis in terms you can reasonably understand. When it is not medically advisable to give you such information, the information will be given to an appropriate person on your behalf. You have the right to know, by name, the physician responsible for coordinating your care.

- You have the right to receive from your physician any information neccessary to give informed consent prior to the start of any procedure and/or treatment. Except in emergencies, such information for informed consent should include, but not necessarily be limited to, the specific procedure and/or treatment, the medically significant risks involved, and the probable duration of incapacitation. Where medically significant alternatives for care or treatment exist, or when you request information concerning medical alternatives, you have the right to such information. You also have the right to know the name of the person responsible for the procedures and/or treatment.

- You have the right to refuse treatment to the extent permitted by law, and to be informed of the consequences of your action.

- You have the right to every consideration of your privacy concerning your medical care program. Case discussion, consultation, examination, and treatment are confidential and should be conducted discreetly. Staff not directly involved with your care must have your permission to be present.

- You have the right to expect that all communications and records pertaining to your care should be treated as confidential.

- You have the right to obtain information about any relationship of the eye center to other health care and educational institutions, as far as your care is concerned. You have the right to obtain information regarding the existence of any professional relationships among individuals, by name, who are treating you.

- You have the right to examine and receive an explanation of your bill regardless of the source of payment.

*Adapted from Borover B, Langley T. Patient's Bill of Rights. Office and Career Management for the Eyecare Paraprofessional. Thorofare, NJ: SLACK Incorporated; 1997.

Figure 1-1. Patient and surgical counselor with eye model. (Photo courtesy of Total Eye Care Centers, PC, Levittown, PA.)

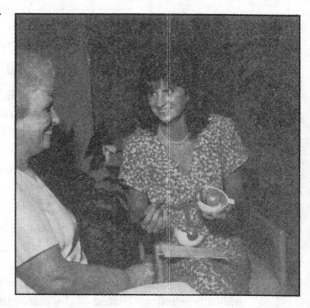

there. Outside discussion during social events regarding patients and procedures performed on them is blatantly unethical. In professional circles, discussion of any case should be solely for educational purposes or in consultation, with careful respect to the patient's identity. Amusing OR events should not be repeated at the expense of the patient.

Chapter 2

Ophthalmic Diagnostic Testing: An Overview

KEY POINTS

- Diagnostic testing provides crucial information required in the preoperative decision-making process, intraoperative course, and postoperative management.

- Diagnostic testing may be used to document the need for surgery.

- Diagnostic testing requires well-trained medical personnel to accurately obtain and perform the various tests.

What the Patient Needs to Know

- These special tests have been ordered by your physician to provide additional information about your eyes.

- You may be required to sign a consent form for some tests.

- While certain tests may require a numbing drop or dilation, the test itself should not be uncomfortable.

- Some insurance companies may not cover certain tests. The insurance clerk may be able to give you this information prior to the test.

Photography

The role of photography in the field of ophthalmology is continually expanding. Subspecialties such as retina and oculoplastics are dependent on clear flow studies and sharp external photography, as these are often used as intraoperative references.

Ophthalmic photography includes, but is not limited to, external and fundus photography, fluorescein angiography, and specular microscopy (endothelial cell counts). Often A- and B-scans are photographed at the time of preoperative study for both chart documentation and later analysis.

Visual Field Testing

Visual field testing (VFT), most often used in glaucoma management, has an integral role in the documentation of field loss in the patient undergoing surgery for dermatochalasis (excess skin of the lids). A preoperative VFT is used to determine whether the oculoplastic procedure is deemed cosmetic in nature. First, the field is run with the patient's lids in their normal, relaxed position. Then the field is repeated after taping the patient's lids up, out of the way. If the dermatochalasis causes a visual field loss, then the taped field test will show an increase in the amount of upper (and sometimes side) vision. In this case, the surgery will improve the patient's visual function (rather than simply his or her cosmesis).

Laser Interferometry

It can be difficult to view the retina or optic nerve through a cataractous lens. This creates a potential problem when attempting to predict a cataract patient's potential vision if surgery were to be performed. Will removing the lens restore the vision to the 20/20 level? Or is there a problem in the "invisible" retina that will only allow a visual restoration of 20/100? The laser interferometer uses a low-grade laser to project a set of lines or stripes onto the retina. The beam bypasses any lenticular opacities, allowing the pattern to be shown directly on the retina. The patient is asked to indicate the orientation of the stripes (ie, straight or tilted to the left or right). Progressively finer stripes are shown until the patient can no longer distinguish their direction. This is converted into a Snellen vision, which is then the "predicted" visual outcome if the cataract were removed.

Potential Acuity Meter

The potential acuity meter (PAM) is another instrument that can be used to estimate what a patient's vision might be if a cataract were removed. The PAM attaches to a slit lamp, and projects a tiny Snellen chart between the particles of a cataract and then clearly onto the retina. The patient reads the smallest line of print that he or she is able. This acuity is considered to be the retina's potential vision.

Contrast Sensitivity Testing

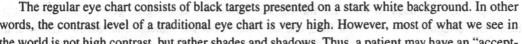

The regular eye chart consists of black targets presented on a stark white background. In other words, the contrast level of a traditional eye chart is very high. However, most of what we see in the world is not high contrast, but rather shades and shadows. Thus, a patient may have an "acceptable" level of vision when tested on the high-contrast eye chart, yet complain that he or she is unable to function visually in an everyday setting. Contrast sensitivity testing (CST) measures the patient's ability to distinguish between various contrasts, and thus gives a more realistic idea of his or her actual visual function. The patient is asked to recognize and interpret a variety of fine, intermediate, or coarse details presented at differing levels of contrast to the background illumination. The surgeon may consider a failed CST as evidence that cataract surgery is warranted, even in cases where the patient's vision on the traditional Snellen chart seems adequate.

Brightness Acuity Test

Any opacity in the optical media has the potential to scatter light, creating glare which generally causes a decrease in the patient's vision. Cataracts are especially noted for this. Furthermore, if a cataract exists in the central part of the lens, bright light causes the pupil to constrict so that the patient is forced to look through the densest part of the opacity. This can be debilitating when driving in a high-glare situation. The brightness acuity test (BAT) is an instrument used to test the glare disability of a cataract patient. First, the patient's vision is checked with the Snellen chart as usual. Then the patient views the chart through the BAT, which introduces a bright light source to simulate bright sunshine. The pupil will constrict as if outdoors. If the patient's vision deteriorates when the glare from the BAT is introduced, a glare disability is considered to be present. If the deterioration is significant enough, the surgeon may consider this grounds to remove the cataract, despite adequate Snellen vision (ie, without the light from the BAT).

A-Scan Biometry

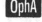

A-scan biometry measures the axial length of a patient's eye in preparation for intraocular lens (IOL) calculation in cataract surgery. This measurement determines the true length of a hyperopic/myopic eye versus a lens-induced refractive error. Axial length measurements should be rechecked if they are less than 22 mm or greater than 25 mm in either eye. They should also be checked if there is a difference of greater than 0.3 mm between the two eyes. The axial length measurement should correlate with the patient's refraction (ie, hyperopes have short eyes and myopes have long eyes).

B-Scan Ultrasonography

Ultrasonography (diagnostic images via sound waves) is used during pregnancy to determine intrauterine abnormalities of the developing fetus. This same technology is used to view the eye so that the ophthalmologist can determine posterior segment abnormalities where visualization is difficult, such as vitreous hemorrhage or cataract. Conditions such as retinal detachment and orbital tumor can be identified or ruled out.

Corneal Topography

Topography is used to visualize the corneal surface by creating a "geographic map." It is based on reflections from the tear film, and uses color codes to indicate changes in curvature. In general, the blue and cool colors indicate a flatter meridian. The yellows and greens indicate a moderate elevation. The deep reds and warm colors indicate the steepest meridians. Preoperative corneal topography is a standard test performed prior to any refractive surgery. It is very effective in identifying early keratoconus and thinning of the central cornea. There are usually two primary features observed with keratoconus: corneal steepening and asymmetry. In refractive surgery, corneal topography is an effective tool that allows the surgeon to evaluate for any postoperative problem with corneal curvature and its relationship to the ablation process.

Corneal Pachymetry

Corneal thickness is measured in units of microns (units of measurements equal to one-thousandth of a millimeter) via pachymetry. Refractive procedures require depth measurement this precise because blade settings are determined from this data. Pachymetry is also used to determine corneal trephination depth (for sizing the donor button in transplantation surgery).

Keratometry

Keratometry is a measurement of corneal curvature. The vertical and horizontal axes of the corneal surface are assessed and measured in diopters. (A diopter is the unit of measurement of the refractive power of a lens.) Keratometry readings (K readings) should be rechecked if the corneal curvature is greater than 47 diopters or less than 40 diopters. Keratometry should also be repeated if the difference in corneal cylinder is greater than 1 diopter between the two eyes or does not correlate with the cylinder in the patient's refraction. K readings are used in calculating the power of the intraocular lens that is implanted during cataract surgery. Corneal topography is used in refractive procedures.

Muscle Balance

Accurate preoperative extraocular muscle measurement in all directions of gaze identifies the muscle, or groups of muscles, that needs to be altered to obtain the desired result in strabismus surgery. It also provides documentation of the existence of the disorder, as well as preoperative information for later comparison.

Schirmer Tear Testing

OphA

A standardized method to assess for tear deficiency is known as Schirmer tear testing (STT). Schirmer test strips are 3 mm by 20 mm filter papers. A single strip is placed into the lower fornix of each eye, at the nasal third of the lower eyelid margin. The patient is instructed to close the eyes for about 5 minutes. A normally functioning lacrimal gland should produce sufficient tears to moisten at least 10 mm of the strip. Decreased tear production causes dryness, foreign body sensation, and burning. This test usually is performed without any topical anesthesia. Schirmer testing may also be performed after instilling one drop of topical anesthetic into the conjunctival sac to eliminate the reflex tearing caused by the filter paper itself. Some patients will have an exacerbation of dry eye following surgery of the eyelids. The STT thus provides a preoperative measurement for predicting this occurrence, as well as providing a reference point if needed.

Refractometry

OphT

Refractometry is the measurement of the eye's refractive error. (This is in contrast to a refraction, in which a licensed individual combines refractometry and clinical judgement to generate a glasses prescription for the patient.) Corrective lenses are used to determine the refractive power. Preoperatively, refractometry is needed to established the patient's best corrected vision (BVA). It is also used as part of the information input needed to calculate the power of a patient's IOL. In addition, the refractive error must be known prior to refractive surgery to guide the physician as to the amount of correction necessary.

Specular Microscopy: Endothelial Cell Count

Specular microscopy, more commonly known as endothelial cell counting (ECC), is performed to examine the endothelium of the cornea. The endothelium is the inner layer of the cornea which is in contact with the aqueous humor. If the endothelium is not in good condition the cornea swells, becomes painful, and loses its transparency.

The specular microscope passes light through a slit aperture into a system of mirrors with a direct light that passes through an objective lens. The tip of the specular microscope applanates the anesthetized cornea. The assistant then adjusts the focusing knob of the cone lens to focus the image of the cornea. The magnification that is reflected from the endothelium and back through the instrument's eyepiece is 200X. The average central endothelium cell count ranges from 1800 to 4000 cells/mm^2 with an average of 2800 cells/mm^2. Cell density decreases with age, indicating continuous cell loss throughout life. The endothelial cell does not have the capacity to reproduce or replace any cell loss, thus endothelial cell loss is permanent. Any type of anterior segment intraocular surgery has a risk of "bumping" the endothelium, causing cell loss (cataract extraction and phacoemulsification in particular). If the ECC indicates a low count or diseased tissue, the surgical approach may have to be changed. In addition, the surgeon can use the ECC to preoperatively assess areas of the cornea to avoid during cataract extraction with IOL implant, because of their low cell distribution. A viscoelastic substance might be used during surgery to minimize trauma to a compromised endothelium.[1]

Table 2-1.
Preoperative Tests

Type of Surgeries	Diagnostic Tests Performed
Oculoplastic surgery	photography, external measurements (exophthalmometry), visual field testing, optional: Schirmer testing
Extraocular muscle surgery	photography, muscle balance
Corneal surgery	corneal topography, optional: pachymetry, keratometry, specular microscopy
Refractive surgery	corneal topography, pachymetry, keratometry, refractometry
Glaucoma surgery	visual field testing, photography of disc
Cataract surgery	A-scan biometry and calculation, refractometry, keratometry, optional: specular microscopy, B-scan ultrasound, PAM, BAT, contrast and sensitivity
Retinal and vitreous surgery	B-scan ultrasound

References

1. Stein HA, Slatt BJ, Stein RA. *The Ophthalmic Assistant.* 6th ed. St Louis, MO: Mosby-Yearbook Inc.; 1994.

Chapter 3

Anesthesia and Pharmacology

- Local anesthetics should not be mixed too far in advance of a surgical procedure as they may deteriorate, compromising their anesthetic effectiveness. Patient discomfort could result, discounting the advantages of performing the procedure under local anesthesia.

- Medication labels and expiration dates should always be checked during preparation and immediately before administration of any drug.

- An important part of preoperative preparation is confirmation of the patient's identity and operative eye before the administration of any drops or ointments.

Ophthalmic Anesthesia

As with all surgical specialties, effective anesthesia is critical to surgical success. In today's ophthalmic environment, local anesthesia (whether topical or regional) is fast becoming a safer standard. Active patient lifestyles and improved surgical techniques have resulted in same-day surgery and the need for quick recovery and visual rehabilitation. Both local and general anesthesia are discussed below.

What the Patient Needs to Know

- Topical anesthesia means that drops will be used to numb your eye.

- Local anesthetic refers to numbing an area by injecting anesthetic.

- General anesthesia means you will be asleep during the surgery.

- Even if you have topical or local anesthesia, you might still have an IV so that you may be given medicine to help you relax.

- It is vital that the physician be aware of any medications you take, even over-the-counter drugs.

- Tell the doctor if you have had difficulty with anesthesia in the past.

Topical and Local Anesthesia

Recent advances have been made in topical anesthetic techniques, eliminating the need for periocular injections. The surgeon considers the patient's age, systemic condition, and emotional status when advising topical anesthesia. Topical anesthetic drops are placed in the lower cul-de-sac of the eye after gentle retraction of the lower lid. Drops should not be placed directly onto the cornea because this might traumatize it. The natural blinking reflex of the lids distributes the drug evenly across the surface of the cornea, regardless of where the drop is instilled. Care must also be taken not to touch the tip of the drop applicator to the skin, eyelashes, or any other part of the eye to avoid introducing any contaminants. Commonly used topical anesthetics include tetracaine 0.5% and proparacaine.

Successful completion of surgery under topical anesthesia requires constant communication with and reassurance of the patient. Patients who are calm, cooperative, and able to follow directions easily are the best candidates for topical anesthesia.

Local anesthesia (non-monitored anesthesia) and local with stand-by (monitored anesthesia supported by an anesthetist or anesthesiologist) are the anesthesias of choice in most ophthalmic surgeries. Local anesthesia may be administered via infiltration (solution injected beneath the skin, conjunctiva, or into Tenon's capsule) or via a regional block (retrobulbar or facial nerve block injections). Patients receiving local anesthesia may have an IV infusion started before the procedure for immediate venous access in the event of any life-threatening situation requiring administration of resuscitative drugs.

Retrobulbar injections are usually performed 10 to 15 minutes prior to surgery, producing temporary paralysis of the extraocular muscles. Local retrobulbar anesthesia is employed in a variety of ophthalmic procedures. The appropriate solution is injected into the base of the eyelids at the level of the orbital margins, or behind the globe in order to block the ciliary ganglion and nerves. A commonly used medication for infiltration anesthesia is lidocaine 1% or 2%. Onset is rapid, duration long, and it diffuses well into the surrounding tissues. Complicated ophthalmic procedures requiring a longer-lasting local anesthetic may employ Marcaine solution 0.25% to 0.75% in combination with lidocaine. To reduce bleeding and prolong anesthesia, epinephrine in a 1:50,000 to 1:200,000 solution may be combined with injectable local anesthetics such as lidocaine. Epinephrine is a vasoconstrictor and should be used with caution in patients with hypertension, diabetes, or cardiovascular disease. Hyaluronidase {Wydase (Wyeth-Aherst Laboratories, Philadelphia)} is a commonly used enzyme that is mixed with anesthetic solutions to increase diffusion through the tissues and enhance effectiveness of the nerve block.

Facial nerve blocks are used to prevent squeezing of the lids during the procedure. Two common methods are the Van Lint and O'Brien techniques. In the Van Lint technique, anesthetic solution is injected into the outer canthal side (above and below) of the orbicularis muscle, where it reaches the ends of the facial nerve. The O'Brien injection technique is given anterior to the center of the ear.

In peribulbar anesthesia, a needle is directed down to the floor of the socket, or up to the roof of the orbit. The anesthetic infiltrates the soft tissue of the globe rather than being placed in the muscle cone itself.

Intracameral Anesthesia

Intracameral anesthesia is a newer method of ophthalmic anesthesia which has been explored in anterior segment surgery since 1995 by Paul Koch, MD. This technique anesthetizes the iris. Following the application of a topical anesthetic, the operative eye receives 0.25 to 0.50 ml of 1% unpreserved lidocaine through a corneal stab incision. Patients are more aware of the intraoperative procedure, but feel no pain or discomfort.

General Anesthesia

General endotracheal anesthesia still has a vital role in certain subspecialties where control over the intraoperative situation is needed, the procedure is of long duration, or where the patient is too young to cooperate under local anesthesia. It can only be administered by an anesthesiologist. In-depth description of this technique is beyond the scope of this text.

Ophthalmic Pharmacology in the OR

OphT

Dilating Drops

OptA

RA

Drops used to dilate the pupil for examination of or access to the interior of the eye are known as mydriatics or cycloplegics. Mydriatic drugs dilate the pupil but permit the eye to focus. A commonly used mydriatic is phenylephrine. A cycloplegic drug dilates the pupil and also prevents the eye from focusing. Common cycloplegic drugs include tropicamide 1%, cyclopentolate 1%, and atropine 1%. Of these cycloplegics, atropine has the longest dilating effect of up to 7-10 days.

Constricting Drugs

OptA

RA

Drugs that cause the iris sphincter muscle to contract and constrict are known as miotics. A commonly used miotic drop is pilocarpine. In ophthalmic procedures requiring rapid pupillary constriction (such as cataract surgery after implantation of an intraocular lens) acetylcholine {Miochol (CIBA Vision Corp., Atlanta, GA), Miostat (Alcon Surgical, Fort Worth, TX)} may be injected intraocularly. Because acetylcholine is relatively unstable as a solution, it is prepared for injection immediately before use.

Antibiotics and Corticosteroids

Antibiotics are most commonly used prophylactically to prevent infection before, during, and after intraocular surgery. Postoperatively, the eye may be patched with bacitracin or neomycin sulfate ointment, which is placed in the cul-de-sac of the lower lid.

Many corticosteroid ophthalmic preparations are available to today's surgeon. They are used to inhibit inflammatory response postoperatively.

Hyperosmotic Drugs

Drugs employed to shrink the vitreous body and reduce intraocular pressure by draining fluid out of the tissues are known as hyperosmotics. Ophthalmic procedures that require lower, controlled intraocular pressure employ these drugs. Commonly used hyperosmotic drugs are acetazolamide {Diamox (Lederle Laboratories, Wayne, NJ)}, glycerol, and isosorbide. The OA should note that by nature these drugs are classified as diuretics and patients should be appropriately counseled about possible increased urination. In addition, acetazolamide specifically is contraindicated in those patients with allergies to sulfa drugs.

Ophthalmic Stains

Fluorescein sodium is a yellow-green dye and topical stain used for diagnostic purposes. Available in both strip and solution form, it is used to stain the cornea to evaluate any disruption of the corneal epithelium. When fluorescein is employed in the OR environment, strips are preferred, as solutions may easily become contaminated and introduce infectious organisms into the eye.

Ophthalmic Viscoelastics

Viscoelastics are thick, jelly-like substances used in intraocular procedures to protect the corneal endothelium. They are made from natural or synthetic sodium hyaluronate {Healon (Pharmacia Ophthalmics, Monrovia, CA), Amvisc (Anika Therapeutics, Woburn, MA)} or combined with chondroitin sulfate {Viscoat (Alcon Surgical, Fort Worth, TX)}. They function as lubricants as well as providing viscoelastic support. In vitreo-retinal surgery they may be used as vitreous replacements.

Antimetabolites

For more information on the definition and use of antimetabolites {5-Fluorouracil and Mitomycin (Bristol-Myers Squibb, Princeton, NJ)} in glaucoma surgery, see Chapter 12, *Glaucoma*.

Ocular Analgesics

Topical non-steroidal anti-inflammatory drugs (NSAIDs) are primarily useful as postoperative analgesics. Prostaglandins are potent, natural, hormone-like substances that are found in the body and formed by the critical enzyme cyclooxygenase. It is this enzyme that sensitizes afferent nerve endings, resulting in ocular pain. NSAIDs block the formation of cyclooxygenase. Common NSAIDs utilized postoperatively by ocular surgeons today are diclofenac sodium 0.1% {Voltaren (CIBA Vision Corp., Atlanta, GA)} and ketorolac {Acular (Allergan, Inc, Irvine, CA)}. NSAIDs cause little, if any, rise in intraocular pressure, which can be a problem when steroids are used.

Chapter 4

Disinfection and Sterilization Techniques

- To insure successful sterilization, ophthalmic surgical instruments must be wiped clean and irrigated thoroughly after use to remove any residual blood or tissue products.

- The two most common methods of sterilization are pressurized steam (autoclaving) or gas (ethylene oxide or EO_2).

- Infection control programs in hospitals and operating rooms must be followed by all hospital personnel.

- Sterilization is the complete destruction of all microorganisms. Instruments are either sterile or nonsterile. *There is nothing in between.*

Infection Control

Effective infection control procedures in the operating room must be followed by all hospital personnel including surgeons, assistants, scrub and circulating nurses, cleaning personnel and anyone else who is in contact with the patient or OR. Infection control is the result of knowing how microorganisms produce an infection as well as understanding their potential for transmission to the wound in the OR environment.

Infectious Microorganisms

Bacteria, fungi, protozoans, algae, and viruses are all living microorganisms that are very tiny and difficult to see with the naked eye. Infections that invade the body systemically can also infect the eye. Proper naming of the various microorganisms is done by shape, staining effect, and culture characteristics through a microscope.

Microorganisms are classified by their names (genus and species) or other indications, such as their shape and means to take up stain (gram positive). Categorization of organisms is necessary to determine treatment course because certain groups respond to specific treatments.

The most common site of staphylococci, gram-positive organisms is the skin surface. Because patients and/or personnel may be carriers of staphylococci, cleanliness of the OR environment, proper handling and sterilization of linens and equipment, and proper hand washing techniques (per hospital protocol) are all crucial in the prevention of infection transmission.[1]

Streptococci have a round shape and are gram-positive. Of these organisms, the bacterium that most frequently affects the eye is *streptococcus pneumoniae*. Conjunctivitis, corneal ulcers, or infection within the eye (endophthalmitis) are known to be caused by this microorganism.

Haemophilus influenzae, Haemophilus aegyptius, Moraxella, and *Pseudomonas aeruginosa* are bacterial gram-negative rods. Of these, *Pseudomonas aeruginosa* is the organism that is most destructive to the eye.

Viruses are the smallest of infectious organisms. The herpes simplex virus can invade the corneal epithelium, causing a corneal ulcer which is dendritic or tree-like in appearance. These corneal surface changes are not often visible through the slit lamp unless fluorescein is applied. Viruses can be transmitted through the oral, respiratory, intestinal, and urinary tracts.

HIV (human immunodeficiency virus) is the virus that causes acquired immunodeficiency syndrome (AIDS). HIV has been detected in amniotic fluid, blood, breast milk, cerebrospinal fluid, saliva, semen, urine, and vaginal discharges of persons infected with the HIV virus. HIV can be transmitted by exposure to blood and other bodily fluids by mucous membranes. One should adhere to specific institutional policy if potential exposure to the virus occurs.

As a healthcare professional, it is necessary to ensure that there is good ventilation in the OR suite and the systems are in good working order. Sterilization of supplies and instrumentation, accurate handling of diseased clothing, and following aseptic techniques (including proper pre-operative scrubbing of the operative site) are methods used in the prevention of infection.

Universal Precautions

Universal precautions are guidelines designed to control the transmission of any infectious blood-borne pathogens. They are not exclusively directed at the control of AIDS. For all invasive procedures, universal precautions should be observed with a basic assumption that all recipients of healthcare could be infectious. This protects not only the healthcare professional, but the patient as well. The Occupational Safety and Health Administration (OSHA) published guidelines on March 6, 1992 regarding exposure to blood pathogens in the workplace. OSHA guidelines state that the best way to reduce transmission of blood pathogens is to reduce the risk of exposure. OSHA policies should be adhered to per hospital and/or ambulatory surgery center (ASC) established policy guidelines.[1]

Disinfection

The goal of disinfection is to reduce the sources of infection. Using chemical solutions is the most common method. There are two solutions used in healthcare settings today—chemical disinfectants and chemical antiseptics. There are some chemicals that can be used for both purposes.

Surgical instruments must be thoroughly cleaned and as dry as possible in order for disinfection to be effective. When sterilization is not possible, high levels of disinfectants should be used on surgical instruments. The various disinfecting agents used today in office settings, hospitals, and ASCs vary according to institutional policy.

Sterilization

Items are either sterile or nonsterile, there is no in between. Microbial life is destroyed by introducing all materials to either physical or chemical treatments. Sterilization is achieved by the complete destruction of all microorganisms and their spores. Of all the living microorganisms, bacterial spores are the most obstinate. Sterilization effectiveness is based on the killing of these spores.[2]

A strict regimen of thorough cleaning and preparation of the microsurgical instruments prior to sterilization is critical. Do not overload the instrument tray, place all instruments in an open position, and make sure they are not touching each another. Further information can be found in Chapter 7.

Common Methods of Sterilization

Steam Sterilization (Autoclave)

There are two basic steam sterilizers—gravity displacement (Figure 4-1) and high vacuum (Figure 4-2). Steam sterilization is the most frequently used form of sterilizing instruments (moist heat under pressure). Heat or steam sterilization is more damaging to stainless steel instruments; however, the sterilization cycle time is less. Moist heat is more destructive than dry heat to bacteria. In autoclaves, microorganisms are destroyed by breaking down protein within the cells.

Under 15 pounds of pressure at 250° F (121° C) requires 15 to 30 minutes exposure time for effective sterilization. Under the pressure of 270° F (132° C), necessary autoclave time is 3 minutes. In general, less sterilization time is required if pressure and temperature settings are higher in the sterilization process.[2]

It is the responsibility of the OA to check the autoclave and verify that it is in good working order, operating in both the steam and drying cycles.

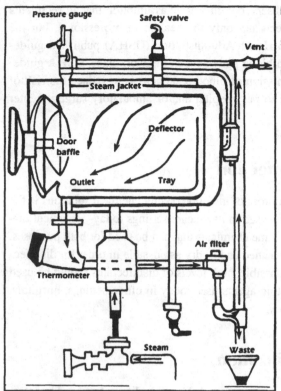

Figure 4-1. Gravity displacement steam sterilizer. (Reprinted with permission from Jackson-Williams B. *Ophthalmic Surgical Assisting*. 2nd ed. Thorofare, NJ: SLACK Incorporated; 1992.)

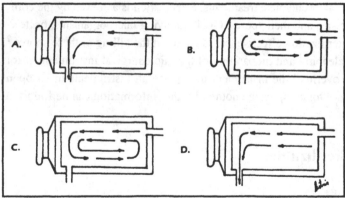

Figure 4-2. A. Vacuum pumps air. B. Chamber and load are heated at high speed. C. Sterilizing cycle is shortened. D. Chamber is evacuated and returned to atmospheric pressure. (Reprinted with permission from Jackson-Williams B. *Ophthalmic Surgical Assisting*. 2nd ed. Thorofare: SLACK Incorporated; 1992.)

Flash Sterilization

High speed sterilization in a conventional autoclave is often referred to as flash sterilization. Flash sterilization should only be used when there is not enough time to sterilize by other methods, and an individual item is needed immediately. Originally, flash steam sterilization was developed for when an item essential to complete the case was dropped or contaminated in an operating room. Usually the temperature is set at 270° F (132° C) under 28-32 lbs of pressure. Flat surface items can be sterilized for 3 minutes; any cannulated or tube-like item must be sterilized for 10 minutes.

Plasma Sterilization

Low-temperature plasma sterilization is one of the most technologically advanced procedures

Table 4-1.
Major Categories of Chemical Disinfectants

Disinfectant	Advantages	Disadvantages	Uses

Alcohol (ethyl or isopropyl)	Fungicidal
	Bactericidal
	Tuberculocidal
	Active against viruses
	Fast acting
	Non-staining
		Non-sporicidal
		Ineffective on evaporation
		Cannot be used on
		  instruments with cement
		  mountings (dissolves
		  cement)
		Inadequate for AIDS virus
			Housekeeping
			  disinfectant
			Used on semi-
			  critical instruments
			  after 0.2% sodium
			  nitrate is added
			Disinfects thermo-
			  meters
			Skin antiseptic

Halogens (chlorine or iodophors)	*Chlorine*
	Highly active as free
	  chlorine in slightly
	  acid solution
	Effective against
	  gram negative and gram
	  positive bacteria
	  and viruses
	Effective against
	  hepatitis virus
	Low cost, toxicity,
	  and irritancy
		Cannot be used on instru-
		  ments (corrosive to metals)
		Non-sporicidal
		Inactivated by organic
		  matter
		Difficult to combine
		  with detergent for
		  single cleaning formula
			Disinfects renal
			  dialysis equipment
			Widely used for
			  disinfection of
			  toilets, lavatories,
			  bathtubs
			Bleach for laundry
			Sanitizer for dish-
			  washing
			Disinfection of
			  hydrotherapy tanks

	Iodophors
	Bactericidal
	Pseudomonacidal
	Fungicidal
	Tuberculocidal
	Virucidal
	Versatile
	Rapid action
	Non-irritating if no
	  iodine allergy exists
	  and is fully rinsed
		Harmful to rubber
		  and some plastics
		May burn tissue
		Inactivated by organic
		  matter
		Corrosive to metals
		  unless combined
		  with rust inhibitor
		May stain fabrics,
		  plastics, and other
		  synthetic materials
			Instrument disinfec-
			  tants after 0.2%
			  sodium nitrate is
			  added
			Thermometers (tinc-
			  ture or iodine or
			  iodophors)
			Disinfecting some
			  kitchen or nursery
			  equipment

Phenols	Bactericidal
	Pseudomonacidal
	Fungicidal
	Lipid virucidal
	Remains active
	  after prolonged
	  drying
		Leaves a film on surfaces
		  (build up must eventually
		  be removed)
		May cause skin irritation
		  and depigmentation with
		  long periods of use
		  (gloves should be worn)
		Non-sporicidal
		Inactivated by organic matter
		Corrosive to rubber and
		  some plastics
			Housekeeping
			  disinfectant
			Used as instrument
			  disinfectant if inst-
			  ruments are not
			  designed for skin or
			  mucous membrane
			  contact

Table 4-1 continued.

Disinfectant	Advantages	Disadvantages	Uses

Quaternary Ammonium Compounds	Germicidal
	Detergent properties
	Cationic surface
	  active compounds
	Wetting agents
	Effective against
	  M. tuberculosis and
	  gram negative bacteria
		Non-sporicidal
		Absorbed and/or neutralized
		  by cotton wool
		Ineffective as skin antiseptic
		Incompatible with soap
		Decreased action in the
		  presence of organic
		  matter
			Housekeeping
			  programs for walls,
			  floors, and furnishing
			Should never be used
			  for disinfecting
			  instruments

Aldehydes	*Glutaraldehyde*
	Bactericidal
	Pseudomonacidal
	Fungicidal
	Tuberculocidal
	Virucidal in alcohol
	Active in the presence of
	  organic matter
	Compatible with metal,
	  rubber, and plastic
	  materials
		Unstable (effective life
		  2 to 30 weeks)
		Some glutaraldehydes
		  may cause chemical
		  burns on skin
		  and mucous membrane
		Contamination is
		  possible during wrapping
		  and drying process
		Alkaline glutaraldehyde will
		  corrode and stain high
		  carbon metals
		Destroys proteins
		Will damage lenses after
		  long periods of use
			Respiratory therapy and
			  anesthesia equipment
			Certain items that
			  cannot be steam or
			  gas sterilized
			Widely used for semi-
			  critical instruments

	Formaldehydes
	  (37% in water, 80% in
	  70% isopropyl alcohol)
	Bactericidal
	Pseudomonacidal
	Fungicidal
	Tuberculocidal
	Virucidal
		Toxic to tissue (must be
		  thoroughly rinsed
		  from instruments)
		Highly corrosive
		Vapor has limited uses as
		  sterilant
		High risk when cleaning
		  hemodialysis systems:
		  toxic to patients and personnel
		Absorbed by porous materials
			Can be used for cold
			  sterilization of instru-
			  ments after adding
			  0.2% sodium nitrate
			Sometimes used to
			  clean hemodialysis
			  water systems

Data from Brooks G. Medical Microbiology. *19th ed. Norwalk, Conn.: Appleton & Lange; 1991. & Soule B.* The Apic Curriculum for Infection Control Practice. *Dubuque; 1983.*

in sterilization. A wide range of microorganisms are destroyed through this process. Low-temperature hydrogen peroxide gas plasma is used to achieve fast low-temperature, low-moisture sterilization in this approach. This type of sterilization may decrease the usage of steam and ethylene oxide sterilization.[3]

Chemical or Cold Sterilization

Chemical agents provide an alternative method of sterilization for instruments and new materials that cannot be autoclaved, or in situations where autoclaving is not available. Cold sterilization also known as chemical sterilization. The minimum time for chemical sterilization is 20 minutes. In some facilities it is procedural policy to add a rust inhibitor to the germicidal chemical solution to prevent instruments from rusting in the pan. In addition, padding should be placed on the bottom of the pan to prevent the instruments from becoming damaged due to metal-to-metal contact. Refer to Table 4-1 for the categories of chemical disinfectants.

Gaseous Chemical Sterilization

The most common form of gas sterilization is ethylene oxide (EO_2). Gas dry chemical sterilization is the least taxing on fragile microsurgical instrumentation. IOL implants are sterilized by this method. Exposure times range from 1 ½ to 2 hours with a temperature range of 50° to 60° and a humidity range of 40% to 80%. It is essential to allow proper cooling time and aeration prior to handling or use after sterilization.[4]

EO_2 sterilization has several advantages. First, it is usable on materials that cannot tolerate other sterilization methods. It is also the least damaging to fragile instruments. EO_2 allows for excellent penetration, and is very effective against all microbes and spores. The disadvantages of this method include the fact that it is expensive and requires special equipment. It also takes longer to achieve adequate sterilization. Finally, the compounds used are toxic and highly flammable.[5]

Liquid Chemical Sterilization

Bacterial and fungal spores, tubercle bacilli, viruses, and all forms of microbial life can effectively be destroyed by liquid chemosterilizers. The most common and effective liquid chemosterilizer is activated glutaraldehyde 2%. For proper sterilization to occur using this method, instruments must be subjected to the liquid chemosterilizer for at least 10 hours. This is not the preferred method of sterilization in hospitals or ASCs today because too much time is necessary to achieve proper sterilization. Aqueous formaldehyde and peroxyyacetic acid are other chemosterilizers not often used today.

Recommended Materials for Packaging

`OphA`

Proper packaging for sterilization is chosen by the type of sterilization method used. Packaging materials should be durable to prevent tearing and puncture (by staples or clips) and should provide an effective barrier against microorganisms. The two common methods of wrapping articles for sterilization are envelopes and peel packs.

Notes:
- Packages are sealed with a heat sealer or heat/gas-sensitive indicator tape.
- Single use items are not meant to be resterilized.
- Allow for adequate penetration and release of gas and moisture for gas sterilization.
- Allow adequate air removal and steam penetration for steam sterilization.[6]

Recommendations for Packaging

`OphA`

- Muslin wrapped items should be double wrapped immediately.
- Manufacturers of packaging materials other than muslin must show data that indicate their products are equivalent to the muslin time temperature profile when steam sterilization is used.
- Polypropylene film (1-3 mm thickness) is the only plastic acceptable for steam sterilization.

- Nylon is not acceptable packaging for gas sterilization.

- Per hospital or ASC, any sterilized package should be marked or labeled with a lot control number that identifies the date of sterilization, sterilization used, and the date of expiration.

- Pack sizes should be no larger than 12 in. x 12 in., no heavier than 12 pounds, and no greater than 7-2/10 lbs per cubic feet in density.[6]

References

1. Meeker MH, Rothrock JC. *Alexander's Care of the Patient in Surgery.* 10th ed. St Louis, MO: Mosby-Year Book Inc.; 1995.

2. Stein HA, Slatt BJ, Stein RA. *The Ophthalmic Assistant.* 6th ed. St Louis, MO: Mosby-Year Book Inc.; 1994.

3. Meeker MH, Rothrock JC. *Alexander's Care of the Patient in Surgery.* 10th ed. St Louis, MO: Mosby-Year Book Inc.; 1995.

4. Jackson-Williams B. *Ophthalmic Surgical Assisting.* 2nd ed. Thorofare, NJ: SLACK, Inc.;1993.

5. Stein HA, Slatt BJ, Stein RA. *The Ophthalmic Assistant.* 6th ed. St Louis, MO: Mosby-Year Book Inc.; 1994.

6. Jackson-Williams B. *Ophthalmic Surgical Assisting.* 2nd ed. Thorofare, NJ: SLACK, Inc.; 1993.

Chapter 5

Preoperative Scrubbing, Gowning, and Gloving Procedures

KEY POINTS

- Preoperative hand scrubbing, gowning, and gloving protocols should be established and regularly reviewed by the individual facility's policy and procedure.

- After scrubbing, sterile gowns and gloves should be worn. This produces an effective barrier which will minimize the passage of microorganisms between sterile and nonsterile areas.

- The front of the gown, from the chest to the level of the sterile field, is considered sterile.

- Nonsterile areas are the neckline, shoulders, back, and under the arms and sleeve cuffs.

- Any item that is not known to be sterile must be considered as nonsterile.

Surgical Clothing

The OR environment is subject to the risk of airborne contamination from outside materials brought in on street clothing such as dirt, germs, and fungi. Therefore, the surgical team changes into special attire (consisting of lint-free materials) to aid in the reduction of these substances (Figure 5-1). Most ORs have designated locker rooms that serve as the transitional area to change from street wear to surgical clothing. Street clothes should never be worn within semi-restricted (OR hallways) or restricted (OR) areas of the surgical suite. Conversely, surgical attire should be confined to the OR environment and not worn outside. In the event that surgical attire must be worn outside the OR, the scrub suit should be covered by a single-use gown with back closure. Upon return, the cover gown should be discarded. Surgical clothing should never be taken home to be laundered. All reusable clothing should be laundered at a facility approved by institutional protocol. Though possibly viewed as fashionable, it is important to remember that OR attire should never be taken home and is the property of the hospital or ASC.

Jewelry such as rings, watches, and bracelets should be taken off or totally confined with the scrub attire, as they may harbor organisms that are not removed during hand washing. Necklaces also could contaminate the front of a sterile gown or drop into a surgical field.

Head Covering

Head and facial hair should be covered when in the area of the surgical suite. This is accomplished by donning a clean, disposable surgical hat or hood that confines all hair and possible dandruff. Ideally, head coverings are put on first, prior to changing into scrub attire, to reduce the possibility of hair or dandruff being shed on the scrub suit. Headgear should not be worn outside the OR suite.

Scrub Suit

Typically, the scrub suit consists of a two-piece pantsuit. The top of the scrub suit should be tucked into the pants. Care should be taken when putting on scrub pants to avoid dragging the pant legs on the floor of the changing area. Nonscrubbed personnel should wear long-sleeved jackets that are buttoned or snapped closed during use. Long-sleeved clothing prevents shedding of skin from bare arms. Closed jackets lessen the possibility of brushing against a sterile field. Should surgical clothing become visibly soiled or wet, attire should be changed to reduce the potential of cross-contamination.

Masks

In the presence of scrubbed individuals or open sterile items (such as instrument tables, equipment, and liquid preparations), high-filtration/fluid-resistant disposable masks should be worn. A mask should cover both the nose and mouth, be placed securely above the nose contour (this will prevent fogging of eyeglasses), and tied snugly behind the head and neck. Only one mask should be worn at a time. A sterile mask is intended to filter droplets projected from the mouth and nose during conversation, coughing, or sneezing. Masks should not be saved from one operation to the next, left hanging around the neck, or tucked into pockets. A hanging mask would expose any trapped bacteria and render them airborne into the OR suite. Proper removal of the surgical mask is done by loosening the ties. Immediately after removal, it should be discarded directly into the appropriate covered waste receptacle. Hands should then be washed and dried thoroughly.

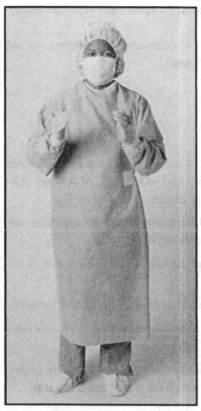

Figure 5-1. Gowned and gloved for the operating room. (Reprinted with permission from Jackson-Williams B. *Ophthalmic Surgical Assisting.* 2nd ed. Thorofare, NJ: SLACK Incorporated; 1992.)

Shoe Covers

Hospital or ASC guidelines will dictate the policy regarding footwear in the surgical environment. Shoes must be covered for sanitary reasons. Shoe covers should be changed whenever they become torn, wet, or soiled, and must be removed and discarded before leaving the surgical area. Upon reentry, clean ones should be put on. Shoe covers are usually found in an area adjacent to the semi-restricted area entrance.

Aseptic Technique

The Association of OR Nurses, Inc. (AORN) has instituted a series of recommended practice guidelines regarding aseptic technique in the operating room environment. These basic guidelines are outlined below and apply to the ophthalmic OR setting, whether it be hospital- or ASC-based.

Surgical Hand Scrub Procedures

Nail polish may chip, crack, or harbor organisms and should be removed before handwashing. Acrylic or artificial nails may also harbor organisms and fungi, and should not be worn by scrub personnel. The skin is a major source of contamination in the OR environment. AORN states that the purpose of the surgical hand scrub is to:
- remove debris and transient microorganisms from the nails, hands, and forearms
- reduce the resident microbial count to a minimum
- inhibit rapid rebound growth of microorganisms[1]

Therefore, all personnel should be in surgical attire before beginning the surgical hand scrub[1]:

all jewelry removed or secured to a two-piece scrub suit consisting of pants and shirt (tucked in), head covering, mask, and shoe covering.

A surgical hand scrub agent, as approved by the facility's infection control committee, should be used for all surgical hand scrubs.[1] According to AORN it should:

- significantly reduce microorganisms on intact skin
- contain a non-irritating antimicrobial preparation
- have a broad spectrum
- be fast acting and/or have a residual effect[1]

Many operating rooms have sinks with elbow, knee, or foot controls. The surgical hand scrub procedure is standardized according to the institution's policy and procedure.[1] AORN has published the following guidelines that should include, but not be limited to, the following.

- Thoroughly moistened hands and forearms should be washed using an approved surgical scrub agent and rinsed before beginning the surgical scrub procedure.

- Areas underneath the nails should be cleaned under running water using a nail cleaner as designated by the facility.

- An antimicrobial agent should be applied with friction to the wet hands and forearms.

- The fingers, hands, and arms should be visualized as having four sides; each side must be scrubbed effectively.

- Hands should be held higher than the elbows and away from the surgical attire to prevent contamination and to allow water to run from the cleanest area down the arm.

- The brush or sponge used should be discarded appropriately.

- Care should be taken to avoid splashing water onto surgical attire as a sterile gown cannot be placed over damp surgical attire. This would result in contamination of the gown by soak-through moisture.[1]

Guidelines for subsequent hand scrubs are determined by an individual facility's policy and procedure.

Surgical Gowning and Gloving Procedures

An auxiliary table is set up with sterile gowns and gloves for both the OA and surgeon. A sterile towel is placed on top of the gown, to be used for careful drying of the hands before taking up the gown. The gown is folded so that the scrub OA can unfold and put the gown on without touching the outer side. Sleeves should have fitted wrists. Sterile water may be available and poured into a basin to rinse any powder off of the surgical gloves. This table should be placed separately from the main instrument table to avoid contamination.

Once gowned, the areas that are considered sterile are in front from the chest to the level of the sterile field, as most scrubbed personnel work alongside a sterile table. Because the arms of a scrubbed individual must move over a sterile field, the sleeves must remain sterile from two inches above the elbow down to the cuff (Figure 5-2). Scrubbed personnel should not let their hands or any sterile item fall below the level of the sterile field.

Nonsterile areas are considered to be the neckline, shoulders, under the arms, back, and sleeve cuffs as these areas collect moisture and are subject to friction, reducing their effectiveness as a microbial barrier. Gowns should be secured appropriately in the back to prevent the sides from flying forward and rendering frontal areas nonsterile, or contaminating the instrument table.

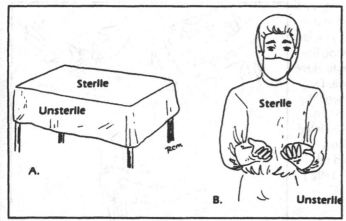

Figure 5-2. Sterile zones. A. Sterile zone confined to the table top. B. Sterile zone confined to waist level. (Reprinted with permission from Jackson-Williams B. *Ophthalmic Surgical Assisting.* 2nd ed. Thorofare, NJ: SLACK Incorporated; 1992.)

Scrubbed personnel should not sit or lean against nonsterile surfaces. However, scrubbed personnel may be seated when the entire surgical procedure is performed at that level.

There are two basic sterile gloving techniques. The closed gloving technique is considered the best method as it reduces the possibility of contamination. In this technique, the scrub OA slides his or her hands into the sleeves of the gown until the cuffs can be grasped between the fingers and thumbs. The hands do not protrude beyond the gown. The gloves are then laid out on the table with the gown-covered hand. The glove is placed thumb down on the sleeve, with the fingers pointing toward the shoulder. The cuff of the glove is then grasped by the thumb and forefinger inside the sleeve and pulled down completely over the gown cuff. For the opposite hand, the gloved hand simply picks up the remaining glove and follows the same procedure.

Open gloving is performed by picking up the sterile glove by the inside cuff with one hand. Care is taken not to touch the glove wrapper with bare hands. The glove is slid onto the opposite hand with the cuff down. Then, using the partially gloved hand, the fingers are slid into the outer side of the opposite glove cuff (Figure 5-3).

When gloving another, the scrub OA (who is already gloved) widely opens the sterile glove for the surgeon or additional scrub person to insert his or her hand into, pulling the glove over the cuff of the gown (Figure 5-4).

After donning, gloves should be inspected for any holes or tears. Contaminated or damaged gloves should be changed. Preferably, the OA would be re-gloved by another member of the sterile surgical team. Some surgeons may elect to double-glove (wear two pairs of gloves) during certain procedures that may pose a risk of accidental contamination, as in manipulating a nonsterile section of the microscope. Double-gloving would need to be done in accordance with facility protocol and procedure.

When permanently exiting the sterile field, either during or at the end of the case, proper technique should be used to remove the gown and gloves. The gown is removed before the gloves by pulling downward from the shoulders, with the sleeves turning inside-out as the gown is pulled off of the arms. The gloves are then turned inside-out and removed (Figure 5-5).

Figure 5-3. Open gloving procedure. A. Pick up glove by its inside cuff with one hand. B. Slide the glove onto the opposite hand with cuff down. C. Using gloved hand, slide fingers into the outer side of the opposite glove cuff and slide the hand into the glove. D. Slide the hand into the glove and unroll the cuff. E. Slide fingers under the outside edge of the opposite cuff and unroll it. (Reprinted with permission from Jackson-Williams B.*Ophthalmic Surgical Assisting.* 2nd ed. Thorofare, NJ: SLACK Incorporated; 1992.)

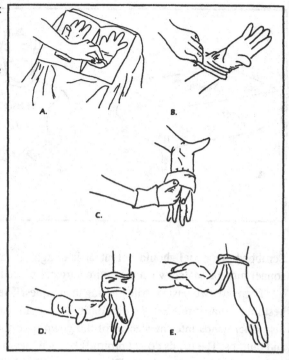

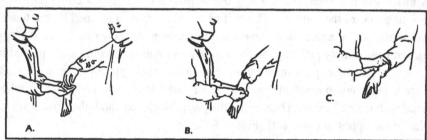

Figure 5-4. Gloving another. A. Spread fingers under glove cuff to create a wide opening. B. Surgeon slides hand into glove. C. Release glove by unrolling it over the wrist and cuff. (Reprinted with permission from Jackson-Williams B. *Ophthalmic Surgical Assisting.* 2nd ed. Thorofare, NJ: SLACK Incorporated; 1992.)

Figure 5-5. Removing gloves. A. Grasp edge of glove. B. Unroll glove over hand. C. Using bare hand, grasp opposite cuff on inside surface. D. Invert glove over hand and remove. (Reprinted with permission from Jackson-Williams B. *Ophthalmic Surgical Assisting.* 2nd ed. Thorofare, NJ: SLACK Incorporated, 1992.)

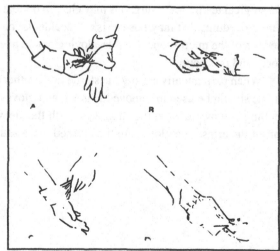

Common Errors in Aseptic Technique

- Mask that covers only the mouth and not the nose.

- Masks that are not tied securely.

- Hair protruding from surgical caps.

- Long fingernails.

- Allowing run-off from the hands instead of the elbows during the surgical scrub.

- Short scrub time and lack of systematic scrub routine (must adhere to institutional policy).

- Splashing water onto scrub clothing. This contaminates sterile clothing donned in the OR.

- Using wet towels to dry scrubbed areas.

- Allowing towels to touch nonsterile clothing.

- Contaminating sterile clothing by brushing against nonsterile objects in the OR.

- Holding gloved hands against the body while waiting.

Reference

1. *Standards and Recommended Practices.* Denver, CO: Association of Operating Room Nurses, Inc; 1996.

Chapter 6

Operative Setup, Ophthalmic Draping, and Sterile Technique

- Since most ophthalmic surgical procedures are performed on a conscious patient, the OA should tell the patient what is being done and what to expect, even during the skin prep stage.

- The surgical team is comprised of scrubbed and circulating personnel. Personnel who scrub their hands, arms, and change into sterile gowns and gloves are scrubbed. Those who coordinate the room activities, interface with the patient, and provide support and supplies to the scrubbed personnel are circulators.

- It is the responsibility of every individual on the ophthalmic surgical team to monitor and preserve asepsis and to initiate corrective action when a sterile field has been violated.

Preoperative Setup

Preoperative setup starts with the selection of the supplies and instruments needed for the day's procedures. It is not advised to prepare sterile setups and cover them with sterile sheets too far in advance of procedures. The sterility of an "unguarded" tray is often broken. In addition, removal of the cover sheet may be difficult and cause contamination of the field. Sterile setups should be prepared as close as possible to the scheduled procedure time according to individual institutional policy.

Preparation Table Setup and Patient Skin Preparation

A preparation table, or "prep" table, is assembled with the necessary solutions and supplies needed to prepare the skin and injection of a local anesthetic. It is comprised of antiseptic {Betadine (The Purdue Frederick Co., Norwalk, CT)} and irrigation solutions, gauze, applicators, and appropriate anesthesia solutions, needles, and syringes. It is set separately from the main instrument table and immediately taken away once the anesthetic has been given and the eye prepared.

Double-check that the patient's hair and head are adequately covered with a disposable cap. Skin prep around the operative eye is performed using an alternating technique of painting the skin with the antiseptic solution and washing it off with sterile water. This is done starting with the eyelids, progressing to the forehead, and finishing with the nose. An ever-widening circular pattern is employed. Remember to always work from the inner to outer canthus. The OA should not allow any of the antiseptic solution to enter the eye. The final step is to tilt the patient's head to the side, where the eye is then flushed with sterile saline or water (using a irrigating bulb syringe) into a curved emesis basin placed alongside the face.

Back Table Preparation

The back table consists of the necessary towels, gowns, and gloves needed for the surgeon and scrub personnel. It also contains the drapes for the patient. Basins for solutions and waste are kept here. The main instrument set is placed here for instruments to be picked up and transferred to the mayo stand. Additional gauze, applicators, sponges, and sutures are placed here until needed.

Handling of Suture Materials

Most ophthalmic sutures are packaged with an outside packet that contains an inner, sterile packet. The circulating OA, in practicing sterile technique (Figure 6-1), delivers the sterile inner packet to the sterile field without touching it or allowing it to touch nonsterile surfaces. The inner sterile packet can be removed with the use of a sterile instrument by the scrub OA, or it can be dropped (not tossed) onto the sterile mayo stand or table by the circulating OA. Tossing items onto a sterile field can cause them to roll off the side or knock off other sterile items. Care must be taken by the circulating OA not to contaminate the table by extending his or her arms over the sterile area.

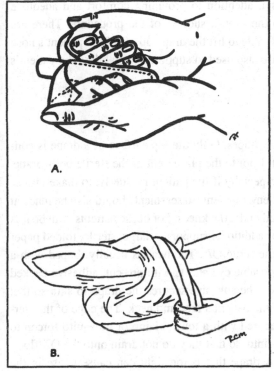

Figure 6-1. Sterile package delivery technique. A. The peel-back method. B. The hand-held method. (Reprinted with permission from Jackson-Williams B. *Ophthalmic Surgical Assisting.* 2nd ed. Thorofare, NJ: SLACK Incorporated, 1992.)

The Mayo Stand

This instrument (mayo) stand is the tray closest to the operative site on which the instruments are arranged to correspond with a particular segment of the procedure. It should be kept organized and uncluttered. Extra instruments, or those needed later in the case, should be arranged on the back table.

Auxiliary Equipment Preparation

Before the procedure begins, circulating personnel should set up, prime, test, and position any auxiliary equipment required to complete the procedure. The phacoemulsification machine, vitrectomy unit, foot pedals, bipolar cautery, overhead light sources, and operating microscope are the types of equipment that need to be adjusted and prepared ahead of time. Foot pedals should be protected from irrigating fluids by plastic covers, especially in cataract and retina procedures.

Patient Positioning and Sterile Ophthalmic Draping Procedures

Most ophthalmic surgical cases are performed with the patient in the supine (flat) position with the head cradled in a supportive headrest. Retinal surgery, however, may dictate various OR table positions depending on the area being repaired. The need for unconventional positions is communicated to the circulating personnel by the surgeon.

Anesthesia, whether local or general, is usually administered before commencement of the draping procedure. When using local anesthesia, attention to providing comfort and adequate breathing space for the patient is important to the overall success of the procedure. There are devices available that can be attached to the OR table to lift the drape up off of the patient's nose and mouth. Doughnut-shaped foam headrests are also used to support and stabilize the patient's head during the surgical procedure.

Body, Head, and Eye Draping

A sterile field is created by the use of sterile drapes. Only the top surface of a drape is considered sterile; the sides and underneath are not. Prior to the placement of the sterile body drape, a warm blanket may be placed over the body, especially if the patient is elderly, to make him or her more comfortable in a sometimes chilly OR environment. Assessment should also be made at this time to see if any additional support is needed under the knees. For obese patients, arm boards on either side of the OR table may be needed for additional support. A large, sterile, folded paper drape is then placed on the patient's body by the scrub OA. The head is usually draped with a double-thickness towel. Most surgeons use disposable eye sheets with pre-cut, adhesive-backed apertures that are placed over the operative eye. The adhesive secures the drape to skin so that irrigating solutions do not run down the side of the patient's face and neck. The edge of the sterile plastic eye drape may be brought up and secured with a towel clamp or mosquito forcep to create a pocket for irrigating solutions to empty into, so that they do not drain onto the OR floor. The eye drape should be snug, but not tight. A drape that is too tight can cause a rise in the intraocular pressure, which can lead to vitreous loss during surgery.

Notes Regarding the Sterile Field

Utmost caution and care are needed when selecting a method of presenting additional items into the established sterile field so sterility is not compromised. Additionally, when sterile liquids are poured into a basin on the sterile field, the edge of the bottle cap is considered contaminated once the cap has been removed from the bottle. When sterile liquids are poured, the entire contents of the bottle should be emptied or the remainder discarded. Replacing a cap on unused liquid renders both contents and bottle nonsterile.

An important rule to remember is "sterile to sterile" and "nonsterile to nonsterile". This means that scrubbed personnel and sterile items contact only sterile areas, and circulating personnel and nonsterile items touch only nonsterile areas.

To maintain the integrity of the sterile field, when scrubbed personnel need to change positions during the procedure they should cross face-to-face or back-to-back. Circulating personnel do not walk between two sterile fields.

Intraoperative Tips and Techniques

- For ophthalmic surgical techniques requiring the use of a microscope, the scrub OA should monitor each step of the procedure through either the assistant scope or closed-circuit television, if available.

- A properly passed instrument is handed to the surgeon so that it is ready to be used without turning or adjusting. As a rule, forceps should be ready to grasp and scissors and knives ready to cut.

- Remember, the attention of the scrub OA should be focused on the procedure at all times. Social conversations not only distract the assistant, but the surgeon as well.

Ophthalmic Sutures and Needles

As an adjunct to this chapter, we feel it is important to include a basic summary of the types of suture material that may be used for a particular surgical case. Keep in mind that the type of case and the surgeon's preference dictate the kind of suture/needle combinations indicated.

Types of Suture Materials

There are several types of suture materials available for use by the ophthalmic surgeon. Each suture possesses unique qualities and is chosen for particular functions during the surgical procedure. Suture material used in ophthalmic surgery is either nonabsorbable or absorbable.

- Plain surgical gut or plain catgut—This suture type is absorbable, eliminating the need for removal. Plain surgical gut is made from the raw material of sheep and beef intestines. Absorption times vary. A reaction to the material may occur, resulting in the formulation of a suture granuloma that sometimes has to be surgically removed. Available in sizes 4-0 through 6-0.

- Vicryl (Ethicon, Inc., Somerville, NJ)—Also known as Dexon (Sherwood-Davis & Geck, Madison, NJ), this is a synthetic suture of greater strength than plain surgical gut. There is less tissue reaction and it is also absorbable. Available in sizes 4-0 through 10-0 (noncoated).

- Silk—An easily handled suture material, it is composed of the raw silk of the silkworm. It is available in a variety of sizes.

- Nylon (DuPont Nylon Intermediates and Specialties, Wilmington, DE)—A strong, synthetic suture material that does not irritate tissues or support bacterial growth. Nylon suture is available in a variety of sizes; the finest (10-0 and 11-0) are used in anterior segment and corneal procedures.

- Polypropylene—Also known as Prolene (Ethicon, Inc., Somerville, NJ), this is a strong, inert suture that is not degraded or weakened by tissue enzymes or time. It is not absorbed. Inflammatory reaction is minimal. Available in sizes 5-0, 9-0, and 11-0.

- Mersilene (Ethicon, Inc., Somerville, NJ)—Mersilene is a polyester fiber suture used in corneoscleral closure. It is stronger than nylon, yet less elastic. It is not biodegradable. Available in sizes 4-0 through 6-0.

Ophthalmic Suture Needles

Needles that are attached to the ends of the above-mentioned suture materials come in a wide variety of lengths, shapes, points, and curvatures, each used for specific tasks during the surgical procedure (Figures 6-2, 6-3, and 6-4).

Figure 6-2. Needle components. (Reprinted with permission from Jackson-Williams B. *Ophthalmic Surgical Assisting.* 2nd ed. Thorofare, NJ: SLACK Incorporated; 1992.)

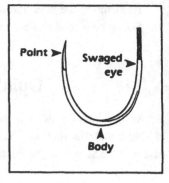

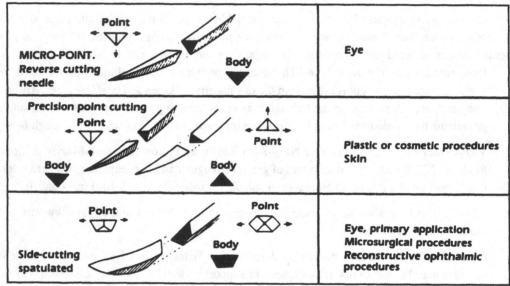

Figure 6-3. Ophthalmic needle points and body shapes with typical applications. (Reprinted with permission from Jackson-Williams B. *Ophthalmic Surgical Assisting.* 2nd ed. Thorofare, NJ: SLACK Incorporated; 1992.)

Figure 6-4. Ophthalmic needle body shapes. (Reprinted with permission from Jackson-Williams B. *Ophthalmic Surgical Assisting.* 2nd ed. Thorofare, NJ: SLACK Incorporated; 1992.)

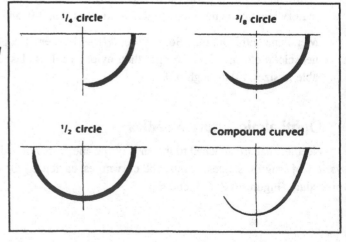

Chapter 7

Handle with Care: Microsurgical Instrument Preparation

- Ophthalmic microsurgical instruments are an investment on the part of the ophthalmologist, hospital, or ASC.

- All microsurgical instruments should be inspected under the microscope.

- Scissors with bent tips, forceps with misaligned jaws, and instruments with surface breaks should all be removed from the surgical set for repair and/or replacement.

- Sterilizing an instrument is not the same as cleaning it. Used instruments must be thoroughly wiped and flushed clean with demineralized/sterile water.

- Never use saline for rinsing instruments because the salt content will adhere to the surface and result in instrument corrosion, increasing rusting or deterioration of the metal.

- Dried blood, tissue, and saline disrupt the integrity of the sterilization process.

- OR personnel who handle instruments should know the name and purpose of each instrument, as well as how to maintain them.

Table 7-1.
Basic Instrumentation

Instrument Type	Function	Description
Forceps	Used to grasp tissue, suture, tubing	May be toothed or smooth; teeth vary in size (0.12 to 0.5 mm); curved, bent, or straight
Scissors	Used to cut tissue, suture	Blunt or sharp; curved or straight; locking or non-locking
Needleholders	Used to hold suture needles	Micro or large; locking or nonlocking
Hooks	Used to identify muscles, grasp IOL loops	Straight or smooth; hooked
Probes/Dilators	Used in lacrimal surgery to open obstructed canals	Vary in size and diameter
Clamps	Used in lid surgery to isolate sections or lesions for excision; create hemostasis	Vary in size and plate diameter
Calipers	Used to measure distances	In ruler or compass form
Cannulas	Used to deliver fluids and substances	Straight, curved; varying surface finishes and gauges
Speculum	Used to separate/hold eyelids	Wire or adjustable; varying size

Types of Ophthalmic Instruments and Their Use

There is an ever-increasing variety of microsurgical instrumentation available to the ophthalmic surgeon. Table 7-1 is a review of some basic instruments and their primary function.

The illustrations in Figure 7-1 represent tips commonly seen on microsurgical instruments for ophthalmology.

Instrument Material Types

Stainless Steel

Stainless steel is the material most widely used in microsurgical instrumentation. Its composition makes it extremely resistant to staining and corrosion. Unlike its name, "stainless" steel only stains less than other metals and is still subject to corrosion.

Titanium

Titanium is a metallic element (symbol Ti) that is found in small quantities in many minerals and is used to toughen steel alloys. Many ophthalmic microsurgical instruments are being crafted of this metal because it is not only strong, but durable.

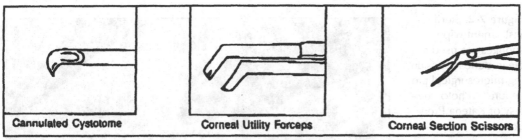

Figure 7-1. Cannulated cystotome, corneal utility forceps, and corneal section scissors (Illustration courtesy of METICO.).

In addition to standard policy and procedure for the care of microsurgical instruments, there are several procedures unique to the care of titanium metal. Use of hydrogen peroxide is not advised, as it may discolor titanium instruments. Brushes softer than facial tissue are recommended to clean handles and instrument tips. Ultrasonic cleaning is not recommended; however, if ultrasound is used do not clean for more than 3 minutes and use only low-powered cleaners. Finally, carefully wipe the surface with an alcohol wipe to restore the original blue titanium luster.

Care and Cleaning

OphA

As with fine jewelry, ophthalmic instruments must be treated with tender loving care. Careful cleaning will insure a long and useful lifespan. In addition to basic care, a routine preventive maintenance schedule should be established for sharpening, realigning, and adjusting. Instruments kept in good condition are less expensive than buying replacements.

To guard the precision tips of instruments during routine handling and storage, it is recommended that the tips be covered with protective silicone tip guards or tubing while they are not in use. (Plastic or rubber protectors may melt and/or shrink around the instrument during the high heat of the sterilization process, most likely resulting in irreparable damage.)

Immediately after surgery and prior to the sterilization process, hand-held instruments such as scissors, forceps, muscle hooks, and needleholders must be meticulously rinsed and wiped clean of residual blood, tissue, or intraocular substances (Figure 7-2). This should be done with lint-free cloths and a mild soap solution. As most ophthalmic instruments have fine surface finishes, the use of abrasive powders, chemicals, or steel wool is not recommended. Cannulas and tubing that have been utilized to deliver or extract fluids, viscous substances, and/or medications must be forcefully flushed clear. This is easily accomplished with clean syringes filled with sterile or demineralized water. Though much connective tubing today is disposable, the silicone connections are not to be ignored as areas where organisms can possibly live. Before clean instruments are returned to the surgical tray, they should be dried completely with a lint-free cloth.

Ultrasonic Cleaning

Ultrasonic cleaning is a gentle method that utilizes ultrasonic wave movements to dislodge any remaining debris that may have settled into minute areas of a microsurgical instrument. These energy waves create tiny bubbles which then collapse, creating a negative pressure that pulls debris away from instrument surfaces. This process is known as cavitation. Ultrasonic cleaning also aids in the breakup of any obstruction that cannot be cleared manually from needles and cannulas. It is recommended for all stainless steel instruments at the end of the day of surgery.

Figure 7-2. Sterile instrument wipe sponges are used to clean delicate tips du ing microsurgical pro cedures. (Photo courtesy of Katena Products, Inc.)

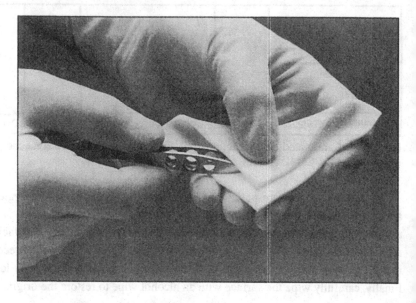

Chrome-plated instruments should not be cleaned ultrasonically because this can loosen the chrome from the base metal underneath. Dissimilar metals such as stainless steel and titanium should not be ultrasonically cleaned together.

Generally it is recommended that fine instruments be placed one at a time in a wire basket without touching each other to avoid damage to tips. Box locks should be opened, and instruments with removable parts should be disassembled. The basket is then suspended in the ultrasonic cleaning solution. After a cleaning cycle of approximately 5 minutes (possibly longer depending on the amount of debris), they should be thoroughly rinsed under running water. Instruments should be bathed in an instrument lubricant or milk after ultrasonic cleaning. To arrest the growth of bacteria in a lubricant wash, only antimicrobial, water-soluble solutions should be used and manufacturer's instructions should be followed. Final rinsing with demineralized/distilled water and drying completes the process before returning them to storage or autoclaving. (Although ultrasonic cleaning removes most debris, it does not negate the need for sterilization.)

Care and Handling of Diamond Knives

Diamond knives used in refractive procedures require specific care and handling. Removal of debris and protection from damage are especially vital to the performance of these tools.

Diamond knives are made from gem-quality diamonds—the hardest element known. The edges are extremely thin and sharp. The blades should never be touched by metal surfaces. Handling and passing the knife in a closed position will help to prevent damage. It is recommended that a rest of some type be utilized when laying an extended blade on the mayo stand so it is not resting directly on the surface.

After use, the diamond blade should be flushed immediately with sterile distilled water squirted with force through a clean syringe. Saline is not recommended. Any dried debris or blood left on the diamond surface will cause a build-up, resulting in the knife's "dragging" on delicate tissues.

Instrument manufacturer METICO (Akorn Inc., Abita Springs, LA) suggests the use of a diamond knife cleaning block to complete the cleaning of the diamond. The block should be moistened at one end with two or three drops of water. Hold the block in one hand and pierce it sever-

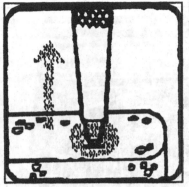

Figure 7-3. Diamond knife cleaning block showing use. (Illustration courtesy of METICO.)

al times with the blade using an up-and-down motion (Figure 7-3). Repeat this process using the dry end of the block, again, very carefully and vertically.

If a cloudy film is noticed on the diamond blade after extended use and/or improper cleaning, place the knife (*always* with the blade retracted into the handle) into an ultrasonic cleaner as described previously. Immerse the knife for 2 hours and complete the cleaning by using the cleaning block.

Keep in mind, this is a gem diamond and when clean, diamonds sparkle. A diamond knife blade is no exception. To remain this way it must continually be protected from damage and kept clean. When the diamond is not cleaned properly before autoclaving, the debris is "baked" on the diamond surface.

Diamond and ruby blades can be sterilized by all conventional sterilization (gas or steam) methods. Ultrasound is not recommended for sapphire blades. Immersion in acetone is not advised for any gem-quality blades.

Instrument Storage

`OphA`

Modern storage cases are designed to be used during the sterilization process as well. These are typically lined with soft silicone mats with flexible prongs which securely hold and separate the array of instruments that form a particular set. The lid and base of the case, as well as the mats, are perforated to allow drainage after rinsing or steam sterilization (Figures 7-4A and 7-4B). Specially designed cases are also available to store/sterilize cannulas. Instruments with curved or angled tips should be placed into the tray with tips pointed downward.

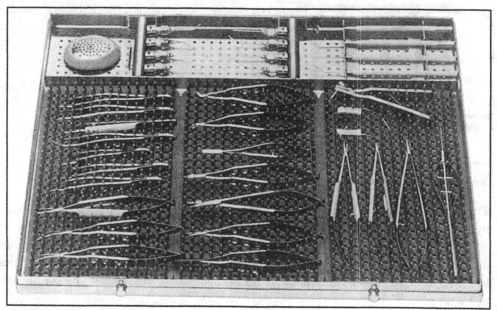

Figure 7-4A. Instrument caddy. (Photo courtesy of Katena Products, Inc.)

Figure 7-4B. Removable lid. (Photo courtesy of Katena Products, Inc.)

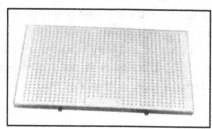

Chapter 8

Oculoplastics: Lids, Lacrimal System, and Removal of the Eye

KEY POINTS

- The oculoplastic surgical candidate may present from a trauma-induced injury or may be seeking a desired cosmetic result.

- Oculoplastic surgery may also be performed to improve visual function.

- Preoperative photography, measurements, and patient expectations are essential elements that contribute to overall surgical success.

The Eyelids: Conditions and Surgical Repair

Ptosis and Dermatochalasis

Ptosis is a condition in which the upper eyelid margin is lower than normal. Ptosis may be congenital, traumatic, age-related, or the result of a systemic condition such as myasthenia gravis (MG). Surgical correction is accomplished by resection (or shortening) of the levator, the eyelid muscle that controls opening and closing of the lid. Approaches are made from the under surface of the eyelid or through the skin. If the levator muscle is paralyzed, it may be necessary to suspend it from the brow muscles.

Surgical repair of the lids may be performed to remove excess skin (dermatochalasis), excise herniated fat pads that extrude from within the orbit, correct problems related to trauma, or to achieve a desired cosmetic result. Surgery for ptosis may also include raising a lid margin that bisects the pupil, thus causing a secondary field defect. In dermatochalasis, the excess skin may overhang the lid margin and obscure vision. In both instances, field defects are documented by visual field testing. This is first performed with the lids in their natural position and repeated with the lids manually elevated. Holding the lids up to the normal position usually resolves the visual field defect and simulates the surgical effect.

Operative Procedure: Combined Upper Lid Ptosis Repair & Blepharoplasty

The patient is brought to the OR and identified by both the attending surgeon and OA. Local anesthesia consisting of lidocaine 2% mixed with epinephrine (9:1 concentration) and Wydase is prepared by the OA. This is passed to the surgeon, who injects it transcutaneously and transconjunctivally to both upper eyelids. The full face is prepped and draped in the usual sterile fashion. The OA passes the marking pen to the surgeon for the upper eyelid creases to be marked and the excess tissue identified. (Figure 8-1)

The OA passes a #15 blade to the surgeon, who incises these marked areas of the right upper lid. The skin flap is raised laterally. A Desmarres eyelid retractor is passed to the surgeon for the lid to be everted, and additional anesthesia is injected transconjunctivally to separate the conjunctiva and Mueller's muscle from the levator muscle. The tissue amount to be excised is marked in millimeters with a #4-0 silk suture from the superior tarsal plate border. The surgeon utilizes a Putterman clamp to incorporate conjunctiva and Mueller's muscle, starting at the superior tarsal border. A #6-0 mild chromic suture is passed through the orbicularis muscle under the skin flap and out through the conjunctiva of the lateral right upper lid. This suture is passed back and forth along the superior tarsal border, and then exited back out through the orbicularis. The tissue in the Putterman clamp is now excised and the suture tied. The remainder of the skin flap is excised, and orbicularis muscle and septum are opened. The fat is identified and removed. Hemostasis is well controlled with a monopolar cautery. The skin is then closed with a running #6-0 mild chromic suture.

A steroid/antibiotic combination ointment is placed in the eye and on the suture line by the OA. Immediate patching is usually not required, especially in a bilateral procedure.

Entropion and Ectropion

The condition where the eyelid rolls inward toward the globe and the lashes rub against the cornea is known as entropion. Surgical correction is accomplished by tightening the underlying

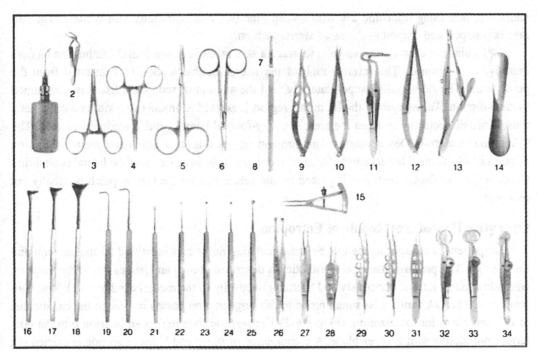

Figure 8-1. A suggested lid surgery set. (Set illustration courtesy of Katena Products, Inc.)

1. BSS Irrigator
2. Towel Clamp
3. Mosquito Forceps, straight (2)
4. Mosquito Forceps, curved (2)
5. Utility Scissors
6. Miniature Blade #69
8. Blade Handle
9. Westcott Scissors, blunt
10. Stitch Scissors
11. Ptosis Forceps
12. Needle Holder, delicate
13. Kalt Needle Holder
14. Lid Plate
15. Caliper
16. Lid Retractor #1
17. Lid Retractor #2
18. Lid Retractor #3

19. Muscle Hook #1
20. Muscle Hook #2
21. Fixation Hook, sharp
22. Chalazion Curette #1
23. Chalazion Curette #2
24. Chalazion Curette #3
25. Chalazion Curette #4
26. Fixation Forceps
27. Conjunctive Forceps
28. Tissue Forceps
29. Fixation Forceps, angled
30. Suturing Forceps
31. Tying Forceps, curved
32. Chalazion Forceps, round
33. Chalazion Forceps, oval
34. Lid Forceps

muscles of the eyelid to roll the lid into position, or by the removal of tarsal tissue from the inner aspect of the eyelid.

Conversely, ectropion is a condition where the eyelid rolls outward away from the globe. This may occur during the normal aging process as lid elasticity is lost. As a result, the inferior portion of the palpebral conjunctiva is exposed. The everted lid is brought back into position against the globe through various surgical techniques.

Operative Procedure: Repair of Entropion

The patient is brought to the OR by the circulating nurse and identified by the OA and the surgeon. Local anesthesia is given transcutaneously and transconjunctivally to the lateral canthus and lower lids using lidocaine 2% with epinephrine (9:1 concentration) with Wydase. The full face is prepped and draped in the usual sterile fashion.

A #15 blade is used by the surgeon to make a skin incision in the lateral canthus, and a canthotomy is performed. The inferior limb of the lateral canthal tendon is disinserted from the periosteum. The lid is pulled superolaterally, and the amount of redundant tissue is determined by the surgeon. The margin of the lid in this region is excised. Conjunctiva, skin, and orbicularis muscle are dissected away from the area. A newly-formed lateral canthal tendon is created. The OA prepares a #6-0 Dexon suture. The surgeon passes this in a horizontal mattress fashion through newly-formed lateral canthal tendon and through the periosteum of the lateral orbital rim. Combination antibiotic ointment is placed on the suture line by the OA. A patch is usually not required.

Operative Procedure: Repair of Ectropion

The patient is brought to the OR by the circulating nurse and identified by the surgeon and the OA. The OA prepares the local anesthetic (as described above) and passes this to the surgeon, who administers it trancutaneously and transconjunctivally to the medial canthus and lateral canthal areas. The OA hands a Bowman probe to the surgeon who passes it through the canaliculus of the lower lids for localization. (Figure 8-2) The surgeon then makes an incision into the posterior conjunctiva with a super blade. A combination of sharp and blunt dissection is carried out to the periosteum of the anterior lacrimal sac. The OA prepares and hands a #6-0 Dexon double-arm suture for the surgeon to pass through the periosteum of the anterior lacrimal sac. Both arms of the suture are also passed through the lateral edge of the medial canthal tendon at its insertion to the tarsus. The suture is tied, and the medial canthus is observed for appropriate position by the surgeon. The OA prepares and hands a #6-0 Vicryl suture to the surgeon, who passes it through the open edges of the conjunctiva and through the lid, exiting out the skin, just inferior to the conjunctival edge of the suture. This is tied to invert the punctum. A lateral canthotomy is performed, and the inferior limb of the lateral canthus tendon is disinserted from the periosteum. The lateral lid is pulled superolaterally, and the amount of redundant tissue is assessed by the surgeon. The OA hands the surgeon Westcott scissors to excise the margin of the redundant tissue.

Conjunctiva, skin, and orbicularis are dissected away from the tarsus and the redundant tissue, and a new lateral canthal tendon is formed. The OA prepares and hands a #5-0 Dexon suture to the surgeon, who passes it through the newly formed lateral canthal tendon and through the periosteum of the lateral orbital rim in a horizontal mattress fashion. The inferior suture is passed over the superior suture and attached to the rim above to the superior suture. This inverts the margin laterally. The suture is then tied by the surgeon. The OA prepares and hands the surgeon a #6-0 mild chromic suture to reform the lateral canthal angle. The skin is closed with a running #6-0 mild chromic suture. A steroid/antibiotic combination ointment is placed on the suture and in the eye by the OA. A patch is usually not required.

Disorders of the Lacrimal System

The lacrimal system consists of the lacrimal gland, punctum, canaliculus, lacrimal sac, and nasolacrimal duct.

The lacrimal gland produces tears. Inflammation of the lacrimal gland is called dacryadenitis. This usually causes pain, discomfort, and swelling in the upper and outer portion of the orbit. Inflammation of the lacrimal sac is called dacryocystitis, which usually causes swelling of the

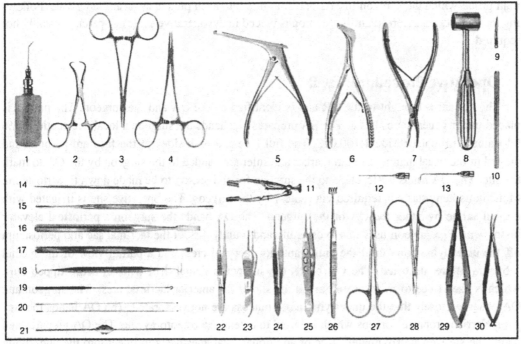

Figure 8-2. Suggested lacrimal surgery set. (Set illustration courtesy of Katena Products, Inc.)

1. BSS Irrigator
2. Towel Clamp (2)
3. Mosquito Forceps, straight
4. Mosquito Forceps, curved
5. Kerrison Rongeur
6. Nasal Speculum
7. Bone Rongeur
8. Mallet
9. Miniature Blade #65
10. Blade Handle
11. Self Retaining Retractor
12. Lacrimal Cannula, straight
13. Lacrimal Cannula, curved
14. Lacrimal Dilator
15. Periosteal Elevator
16. Lacrimal Chisel, straight
17. Lacrimal Chisel, curved
18. Pigtail Probe
19. Retrieving Hook
20. Intubation Set
21. Lacrimal Probe Set
22. Dressing Forceps
23. Tissue Forceps
24. Utility Forceps
25. Suturing Forceps
26. Rake Retractor (2)
27. Stevens Scissors
28. Utility Scissors
29. Needle Holder
30. Stitch Scissors

lacrimal sac. Often, if an infection is present when pressure is applied over this area, pus is expressed through the punctum ("positive reflux"). Chronic inflammation of the lacrimal sac may cause nasal polyps or deviation of the septum, requiring a dacryocystorhinostomy (DCR) to open the nasal canal, allowing unobstructed tear flow.

Operative Procedure: Probing and Irrigation (Pediatric, Under General Anesthesia)

The patient is brought to the OR after being identified by OA and the surgeon, and placed under anesthesia. A punctal dilator is handed to the surgeon by the OA to dilate the upper and lower puncta. The surgeon then prepares to clear any obstructions. The OA hands the surgeon a #00 Bowman probe which is placed through the lower puncta and down into the nasolacrimal duct. This may be repeated on the upper punctum. The OA hands the surgeon a #0 and a #1 Bowman probe which the surgeon inserts one at a time into each puncta as described above. Following the procedure, a steroid/antibiotic drop is placed in the operative eye(s). A patch is usually not required.

Operative Procedure: DCR

The patient is brought to the OR and is identified by the OA and the surgeon. The patient is placed under general anesthesia. The OA prepares and hands the surgeon a local anesthetic of 2% lidocaine with epinephrine 1:100,000. The full face and both sides of the face are prepped and draped in the usual manner. A skin marker and ruler are handed to the surgeon by the OA to mark the site. The OA hands a #15 blade to the surgeon for an incision to be made down to periosteum. Meticulous hemostasis is required via cautery by the surgeon. The operative site is irrigated with normal saline by either the OA or the surgeon. The OA hands the surgeon a periosteal elevator instrument. The surgeon uses this to carefully and bluntly dissect the lacrimal sac and periosteum off the underlying bone until the entire anterior lacrimal crest and a partial view of the medial orbital wall are identified. The OA hands the surgeon a dental drill with an acorn-tipped burr, which is used to perform an osteotomy at the site of the anterior lacrimal crest. The surgeon and OA observe closely that the underlying nasal mucosa are not perforated. The OA hands the surgeon Kerrison rongeur forceps which are used to extend the osteotomy site. The OA prepares and hands the surgeon approximately 1 cc of additional local anesthesia to inject into the underlying nasal mucosa. The puncta are dilated with a lacrimal dilator, and the OA hands a #00 Bowman probe to the surgeon to identify the blockage. The OA hands a #11 blade to the surgeon for a corresponding incision into the lacrimal sac. The surgeon then makes a similar incision in the nasal mucosa, and flaps are created. The OA hands the lacrimal intubation tube to the surgeon for placement into the inferior and superior puncta. The tubes are brought out through the osteotomy site into the nasal cavity and captured with a retrieving hook. The OA prepares and hands a #5-0 chromic suture to the surgeon. The ends of the tubes are tied together with multiple square knots and attached to the nasal wall. The OA prepares and hands the surgeon a #4-0 Vicryl suture. The anterior lacrimal flap is layered to fit together with the anterior flap of the nasal mucosa using the Vicryl suture. The surgeon then uses the same suture material and puts in multiple interrupted sutures to reapproximate the periosteum. The OA prepares and hands to the surgeon #6-0 Prolene suture. This is used to close the muscle and skin in a overlapping mattress fashion. Benzion and Steri-Strips (3M Health Care, St. Paul, MN) are placed over the eye by the OA. Postoperative instructions are sent to the recovery room directing the patient to apply an antibiotic ointment to the area. Continuous ice packs are to be applied to control postoperative swelling.

Enucleation and Evisceration

Enucleation involves removal of the entire globe. Evisceration preserves the scleral shell and removes only the orbital contents.

These procedures are done in the presence of tumor, injury, and severe pain resulting in dysfunction of the eye. General anesthesia is often indicated due to the psychological trauma of removing an eye. (Figure 8-3)

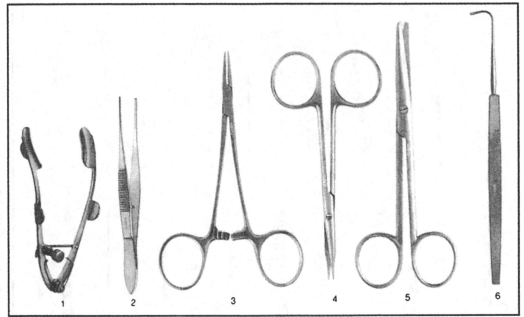

Figure 8-3. Suggested enucleation surgery set. (Set illustration courtesy of Katena Products, Inc.)

1. Speculum
2. Tissue Forceps
3. Mosquito Forceps

4. Tenotomy Scissors
5. Enucleation Scissors
6. Muscle Hook

Operative Procedure: Enucleation

The patient is brought to the OR and identified by the surgeon and the OA. The surgeon verifies with the patient which eye is to be removed and general anesthesia is induced. A decongestant drop is placed between the lids of the operative eye to constrict the blood vessels of the conjunctiva. A retrobulbar injection of 3 cc lidocaine 2% with epinephrine (9:1 concentration) and Wydase is given by the surgeon. Approximately 2 cc is also given subconjunctivally to dissect conjunctiva from the underlying tissue around the limbus, and to aid in hemostasis. The full face is prepped and draped in the usual sterile fashion. A protective shield is placed over the opposite eye. A speculum is handed to the surgeon by the OA for placement between the lids. A 360° conjunctival peritomy is performed around the limbus of the globe using Westcott scissors and a blunt dissection is carried out in all four quadrants. The OA hands a muscle hook to the surgeon, and the four rectus muscles are identified with the hook. A #6-0 Vicryl suture is prepared by the OA and passed to the surgeon. The suture is placed near the insertion of each muscle in a double-locked fashion. Each muscle is then severed from the globe. The OA hands cautery to the surgeon upon request to cauterize any bleeding vessels. Further blunt dissection is carried out and the optic nerve is visualized. The oblique muscles are then severed from the globe. The OA passes a forceps to be placed around the optic nerve. The clamped forceps is left in place for several minutes. The OA passes the curved scissors to the surgeon, who severs the optic nerve. The excised globe is placed in preserving medium and sent to the pathology lab for analysis. The forcep is left in place and a monopolar cautery is used to cauterize the stump of the optic nerve. The forcep is removed and manual digital pressure is applied on the orbit to control bleeding and achieve hemostasis. The surgeon measures and selects an appropriately sized implant (typically glass, plastic, or silicone) to fit in the empty orbit. The remaining muscle and tissue surrounding

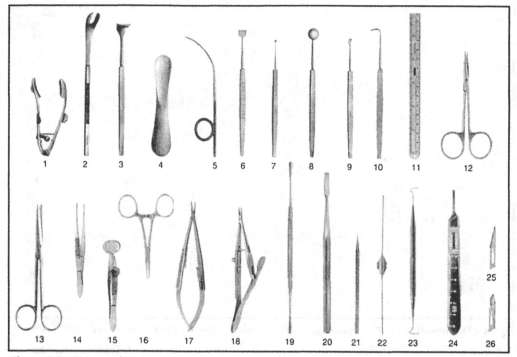

Figure 8-4. Suggested oculoplastic surgery set. (Set illustration courtesy of Katena Products, Inc.)

1. Lester-Burch Eye Speculum
2. Schepens Orbital Retractor
3. Desmarres Lid Retractor #2
4. Jaeger Lid Plate, stainless steel
5. Wright Fascia Needle
6. Knapp Retractor, 4-prong, blunt
7. Meyerhoefer Curette #3
8. Bunge Evisceration Spoon, large
9. Fixation Hook, double, sharp, large
10. Graefe Muscle Hook
11. Stainless Steel Rule
12. Stevens Scissors, standard, straight
13. Enucleation Scissors, medium, curved

14. Tissue Forceps, standard 1x2, straight
15. Francis Chalazion Forceps
16. Hartmann Mosquito Forceps
17. Castroviejo Needle Holder, straight with lock
18. Kalt Needle Holder, delicate
19. Freer Periosteal Elevator
20. West Lacrimal Chisel, straight
21. Wilder Lacrimal Dilator #2
22. Bowman Lacrimal Probe #3-4
23. Pigtail Probe with suture holes
24. Bard-Parker Handle
25. Bard-Parker Blade #11
26. Bard-Parker Blade #15

the implant is sewn over the area with a #6-0 Vicryl suture for movement and support of the future prosthesis. (Figure 8-4) A steroid/antibiotic combination ointment is placed in the cul-de-sac and an orbital conformer shield is placed in the socket. A pressure patch is then applied.

After healing, the patient is referred to an ocularist for fitting of a cosmetic prosthetic shell which will compliment the patient's remaining natural eye.

Extraocular Muscles

- Strabismus, or misalignment of the eyes, affects approximately 4% of children younger than 6 years of age.

- Of that 4%, 30% to 50% will develop secondary visual loss, or amblyopia.

- Early detection and treatment of strabismus is essential in restoring proper alignment of the visual axis, allowing normal development of binocular vision.

- The goal of muscle surgery is to improve muscle function, eliminate diplopia, or improve the patient's appearance and self-image.

Extraocular Muscle Surgery Defined

Our eyes are controlled by six extraocular muscles (EOMs) that surround the eye and attach externally, working in pairs (Tables 9-1 and 9-2). These muscles and their function are illustrated in Figure 9-1.

Strabismus is a condition where both eyes are not focused on or directed at the same object. Because each eye fixates on objects at different points in space, the images received by the brain are not alike. Consequently, the brain is unable to fuse these images, resulting in diplopia (double vision). In children, the brain learns to ignore the unfocused images seen by the deviating eye. Clear sight may develop only in the straight eye, resulting in amblyopia of the deviating eye. Depth perception (three dimensional viewing) will also be lost. Strabismus is classified into the following types: esotropia (eye that turns in toward the nose, the most common type), exotropia (eye that turns outward), and hypertropia (one eye is higher than the other).

EOM surgery is designed to either strengthen or weaken EOMs. These procedures may be indicated in strabismus, when the muscles or their nerves become affected by conditions such as thyroid disease, or when they are entrapped by orbital trauma (as in an orbital fracture). Muscle imbalances are initially identified and then treated with a combination of glasses, therapeutic patching over a period of time, or surgical correction. Not all muscle imbalances are treated by surgical procedures. Esotropias that are caused by excessive hyperopia (farsightedness) may be managed with glasses which reduce or eliminate the strong focusing power of the pediatric eye.

Muscle recession (weakening) procedures are used to move EOMs posteriorly in order to weaken the action of the muscle. To strengthen or enhance the effect of a muscle or tendon, muscle resection techniques are used. Resection procedures consist of moving an EOM forward, shortening it and thus strengthening the action of the muscle. General anesthesia is utilized for the pediatric patient, while adult strabismus surgery is commonly performed under some form of local anesthesia with anesthesia monitoring. Topical anesthetic drops alone (tetracaine 0.5%, proparacaine 0.5%, cocaine 4%) can be used effectively in the cooperative adult patient for certain muscle procedures. If the lid speculum is not spread to the point of pain and discomfort, a lid block is usually not performed. Under all circumstances, discharge is usually the same day.

Fear and the Pediatric Surgical Patient

The OR is not home. Think of how it must appear to a child; the strange masked faces, machines, wires, tubes, lights, and sounds may frighten a young patient. The OA can alleviate some of the apprehension with a warm embrace, smile, and communication. Storytelling can ease a child's concern. A smiling friendly face (even a strange one wearing a mask) can work wonders.

Often a special doll will accompany the child to the OR for a sense of security. The placement of an eye patch on the doll can take the youngster's mind off of his own experience. Even though most muscle surgery is "patch free," this simple action allows the child to care for something that is special to him or her.

Operative Procedure: Muscle Recession of MR (Under General Anesthesia)

After appropriate identification by the attending surgeon, the patient is taken to the OR and placed under general anesthesia. Once placed in the supine position, the patient is prepped and draped in the usual sterile manner to reveal the full face above the nose. (Figure 9-2)

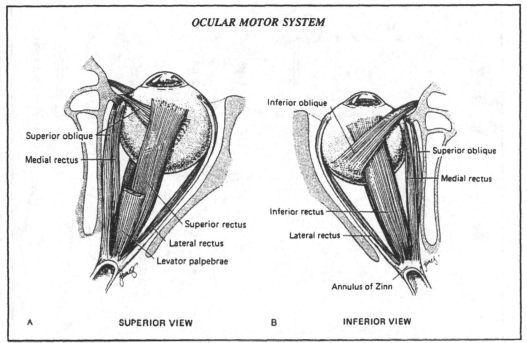

Figure 9-1. Relationships of the EOMs to the eye and orbit. A. View from above. B. View from below. (Reprinted with permission from Rhode SB. *Ophthalmic Technology—A Guide for the Eye Care Assistant.* Philadelphia, PA: Lippincott-Raven Publishers; 1997.)

Table 9-1.
Muscle Abbreviations and Actions

Muscle/Abbreviation	Primary Action	Secondary Action	Tertiary Action
Medial Rectus (MR)	Adduction	None	None
Lateral Rectus (LR)	Abduction	None	None
Superior Rectus (SR)	Elevation	Adduction	Intorsion
Inferior Rectus (IR)	Depression	Adduction	Extorsion
Superior Oblique (SO)	Intorsion	Depression	Abduction
Inferior Oblique (IO)	Extorsion	Elevation	Abduction

Table 9-2.
EOMs Responsible for the Cardinal Positions of Gaze

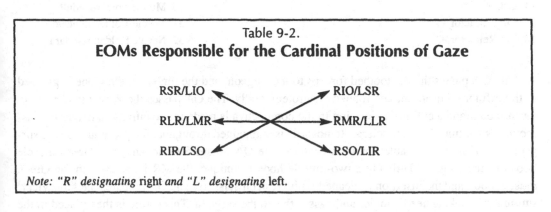

Note: "R" designating right *and "L" designating* left.

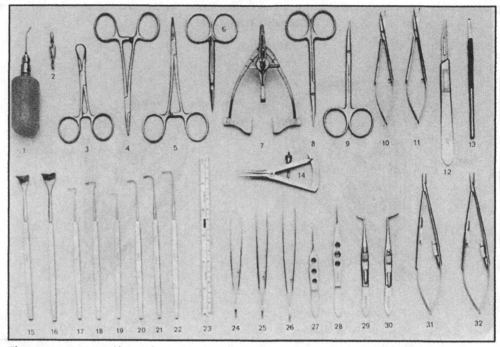

Figure 9-2. Suggested muscle surgery set. (Set illustration courtesy of Katena Products, Inc.)

1. BSS Irrigator
2. Serrefine (2)
3. Towel Clamp
4. Mosquito Forceps, straight (2)
5. Mosquito Forceps, curved (2)
6. Utility Scissors
7. Speculum
8. Tenotomy Scissors, straight
9. Tenotomy Scissors, curved
10. Stitch Scissors
11. Westcott scissors, blunt
12. B-P Handle #3 and Blade #11
13. Beaver Handle and Blade #6900
14. Caliper
15. Lid Retractor #1
16. Lid Retractor #2

17. Jameson Muscle Hook, small
18. Jameson Muscle Hook, large
19. Tenotomy Hook
20. Muscle Hook #1
21. Muscle Hook #2
22. Muscle Hook #3
23. Stainless Steel Rule
24. Dressing Forceps
25. Conjunctiva Forceps
26. Fixation Forceps
27. Tissue Forceps
28. Suturing Forceps, 0.3 mm
29. Muscle Forceps, child
30. Muscle Forceps, adult
31. Needle Holder, delicate
32. Needle Holder, standard

The OA passes the 0.5 toothed forceps to the surgeon, and the limbus of the globe is grasped in the infranasal quadrant and rotated superotemporally. The OA passes the Westcott scissors to the surgeon, and a cul-de-sac incision in the conjunctiva is made in the infranasal quadrant. Dissection is continued to bare sclera. Hemostasis is maintained throughout the procedure by the surgeon, utilizing a disposable hot stick cautery. The OA passes Stevens and then Green muscle hooks to the surgeon. Utilizing a two-muscle hook technique, the MR is isolated on the Green muscle hook and the insertion is cleaned with Westcott scissors. The OA prepares the #6-0 Vicryl suture on a locking needleholder and passes this to the surgeon. This suture is then placed in the muscle just posterior to the insertion, and two locking sutures are placed at the superior and inferior aspect of the muscle. The muscle is then cut by the surgeon from its insertion with Westcott scissors. Calipers are passed to the surgeon by the OA and used to measure the intended amount posterior to the insertion. The #6-0 Vicryl suture is then sewn to the sclera in a crossed sword type fashion at the insertion. The muscle is pulled up firmly against the globe and the sutures are tied securely in place. The OA passes the Westcott scissors to the surgeon who cuts the ends of the suture. The calipers are then passed to the surgeon who uses them to check the placement of the muscle, noting posterior placement to the insertion. The OA prepares the #6-0 plain gut suture on a locking needleholder and passes this to the surgeon. The surgeon sutures the conjunctiva with one interrupted #6-0 plain gut absorbable suture. Again, the OA passes the Westcott scissors to the surgeon who cuts the ends of the suture. The lid speculum is removed from the eye by the surgeon or OA. An antibiotic drop or ointment is placed into the eye by the OA. Usually no patch is applied, as no intraocular surgery has been performed.

Procedure: Muscle Resection of RLR (Under Local Anesthesia)

After appropriate identification by the attending surgeon, the patient is taken to the OR. After being placed in the supine position, the patient is prepped and draped in the usual sterile manner to reveal the full face above the nose.

A lid speculum is placed by the surgeon after several anesthetic drops are placed on the eye by the OA. As this procedure is being done under local anesthesia, a pledget soaked with tetracaine 0.5% is placed on the conjunctiva in the area of the planned incision to insure continued topical anesthesia to the site.

The OA passes the Westcott scissors to the surgeon and a cul-de-sac incision is made in the conjunctiva in the infratemporal quadrant. Hemostasis is maintained by the surgeon with the use of a disposable hot stick cautery. The OA passes two Green muscle hooks to the surgeon. The LR is identified and placed on the two hooks. A caliper is passed to the surgeon by the OA and used to measure the intended amount posterior to the insertion. At this point, the OA prepares the #6-0 Vicryl on a locking needleholder and passes this to the surgeon. Two sutures are placed in the muscle, one in the superior half of the muscle and one in the inferior half of the muscle. Additional locking sutures are placed in each half of the muscle. The OA passes a hemostat to the surgeon, and it is placed just anterior to the suture line to secure the muscle. Westcott scissors are passed by OA to the surgeon to cut the muscle from its insertion. The excess muscle is removed anterior to the hemostat with Westcott scissors. The #6-0 Vicryl sutures are then sewn to the sclera at the insertion in a double "x" fashion (ie, "xx"). The muscle is pulled up firmly against the globe and the sutures are tied securely in place. The suture ends are cut with Westcott scissors. The OA prepares a #6-0 plain gut absorbable suture on a locking needleholder and passes this to the surgeon. This is used to suture the conjunctiva. The lid speculum is removed. Antibiotic drops are placed on the eye by the OA. Usually no patch is applied.

Complications of Extraocular Muscle Surgery

There are a large number of intraoperative and postoperative potential complications associated with EOM surgery. Fortunately, the most severe are uncommon.

Unsatisfactory alignment is the most frequent complication of muscle surgery. Undercorrections are more common than overcorrections. The development of adjustable suture techniques has provided an opportunity to improve the immediate postoperative alignment in certain patients.

Care must be taken by the assisting OA not to tug on the muscles being manipulated during the operative procedure. The oculocardiac reflex, a slowing of the heart rate caused by pulling on the EOMs, can trigger asystole, or loss of heartbeat. Tension on the muscle should be released immediately if the heart rate drops excessively.

Vomiting during the immediate postoperative period is a frequent occurrence that affects about half of all children undergoing EOM surgery. This can be prevented or lessened with antiemetics administered by the anesthesiologist or surgeon during or after the procedure.

Scleral perforation during muscle surgery can be a serious complication of strabismus surgery. Perforation can lead to vitreous hemorrhage, retinal detachment, or endophthalmitis. Cryotherapy over the site may be required to seal the hole.

Sometimes a foreign body granuloma and/or allergic reaction will develop several weeks after surgery, often at the site of the suture. A granuloma is a localized, slightly hyperemic, elevated, tender mass, usually less than 1 cm in diameter. Foreign materials such as eyelashes, cotton fibers, or glove powder may produce the same effect. Granulomas usually respond to topical steroids, but a surgical excision may be required if it persists.

A muscle that is dropped (lost) during the procedure, or a muscle that slips postoperatively, requires immediate surgical intervention to reclaim or to reattach it to the previous surgical site.

Malignant hyperthermia (MH), a rapid rise in the patient's temperature to extremely high levels, is a risk in all general anesthetic procedures, particularly in strabismus repair, and may even be a problem with local anesthesia. Signs of this condition present as tachycardia (accelerated heart beat), tachyarrhythmia (accelerated skipping heart beat), or tachypnea (increased respirations). The surgeon may note muscle rigidity as a first sign. The surgeon may also see darkening of the blood in the operative field, secondary to the increased consumption of oxygen. If this condition is not discovered and reversed, cardiac failure and death usually result. Early detection is essential. Preoperative assessment of previous difficulty with anesthetic agents either in the patient's family or self, notation of elevated serum creatine phosphokinase (CPK) enzyme levels, and intraoperative monitoring of OR temperature are essential. Prompt treatment of this crisis is best left to the attending anesthesiologist. Treatment protocols should be posted in the OR, including aborting the surgery, stopping the triggering anesthetic agent, cooling the patient, and administering dantrolene sodium (a muscle relaxant which should be readily available on the anesthesia cart).

Cornea

- Corneal opacification resulting in visual loss may necessitate corneal transplantation.

- Human cornea tissue is acquired from an organ donor tissue bank.

- Strict maintenance of the sterile field is essential in donor tissue handling during surgery to reduce the possibility of corneal graft rejection.

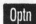

The Cornea Defined

The cornea is the clear, avascular, protective structure covering the front surface of the eye. It consists of five distinct layers: epithelium, Bowman's membrane, stroma, Descemet's membrane, and endothelium. Injury, disease, or inherited conditions may cause scarring, clouding, or distortion. The epithelium, the outermost layer, experiences constant exposure to the environment and is commonly injured by superficial abrasions and small foreign bodies. The epithelium usually regenerates and heals after a few days without residual scarring. The innermost layers of the cornea do not have the ability to regenerate. When these corneal layers are injured, scarring may result as a part of the healing process. When central scarring interferes with vision, depending on the specific condition, a corneal transplant may be an viable option.

Keratoconus

Keratoconus, an uncommon disease process, is characterized by a progressive thinning of the central cornea to a cone-shaped appearance. As the cornea assumes a more conical shape, it becomes increasingly difficult to fit a contact lens that is both comfortable and effective in correcting vision. PKP may be indicated in advanced stages where the corneal apex thins to the point of disruption, in order to restore a cornea of normal clarity and curvature.

Corneal Transplantation

Corneal transplant, known as penetrating keratoplasty (PKP), is a surgical procedure wherein damaged corneal tissue is replaced with donor corneal tissue. Only the central part of the cornea is removed in transplantation, as the corneal limbus of the host is utilized as the site where sutures attach the corneal button from the donor. PKP may either be lamellar (partial thickness) or full thickness. Lamellar PKP is performed to achieve removal of surface corneal opacification where underlying healthy corneal layers exist. Deeper opacification, however, requires the removal of the entire central cornea. "Open sky" is a full-thickness PKP technique where the central host cornea is removed completely, exposing the cavity of the globe. A donor central corneal "button" is placed and sutured down. A technique such as this requires careful monitoring of the intraocular pressure to avoid an expulsive hemorrhage of the ocular contents.

Graft rejection can occur from donor tissue. This complication is minimized by careful preoperative screening and matching of donor tissue to the recipient (Table 10-1). Intraoperative care in handling of the donor tissue and close postoperative follow-up is critical to surgical outcome.

Eye Banking

Human corneal tissue is acquired from an organ donor tissue bank. Donor tissue is usually removed within 6 hours of death. Donor tissue undergoes extensive examination and testing to determine suitability for transplantation (Figure 10-1). The detailed information collected about the potential donor on all the forms illustrated here help to rule out tissue that is unsuitable for transplantation or potentially hazardous to the recovery technician. When serology tests indicate positive results for HIV/1 & 2, hepatitis B, HCV, HTLV-1 (Human T-cell Leukemia Lymphotropic virus) or syphilis, the eye tissue is not used for transplantation. A thorough medical assess-

Table 10-1.
Indications for Corneal Transplantation

Type	Indication
Congenital	
Injury	alkali chemical burns (lye, ammonia)
	blunt, penetrating injury
Infection	*Herpes simplex* virus
	bacterial ulcers
	fungal ulcers
Keratoconus	
Corneal Edema	Fuch's dystrophy (hereditary)
	bullous keratopathy (post intraocular surgery)

ment of the deceased is also performed including cause of death, admitting diagnosis (if applicable), and any recent medical history from the current hospitalization (Figures 10-2 and 10-3). The medical social history is very important. It produces answers to questions not found on a hospital chart. The next of kin are a good source of medical and personal information which is used to determine the acceptability of eye tissue. A physical inspection of the donor is also done to look for lacerations, abrasions, tattoos, ulcers, or signs of IV drug use (Figure 10-4).

Acceptable eye tissue is placed in a preservative medium for transport to a prospective recipient. Techniques now allow for storage up to 7 days postmortem. Therefore, most corneal transplants are scheduled as elective, nonemergent procedures.

The vitrectomy unit is prepared and placed on stand-by status. Scleral support rings, known as Flieringa rings, should be used in all aphakic patients or in phakic eyes in which cataract extraction is anticipated. These rings stabilize the globe during trephination and prevent the collapse of the anterior segment after the removal of the host cornea.

Operative Procedure: Penetrating Keratoplasty

It is important to note if the PKP will be performed on a phakic eye. Unless cataract surgery is anticipated as part of the procedure, the pupil should be constricted preoperatively to help protect the lens.

The scrub OA, after appropriate sterile gowning and gloving, drapes the mayo stand in sterile fashion and organizes the instrument tray. (Figure 10-5) The donor corneal tissue is removed from the transport vial and placed in a container with OptiSol (E.I. duPont de Nemours and Company, Wilmington, DE) storage medium in preparation for the upcoming procedure. The color of the Optisol medium is noted by the OA. (Pink indicates a normal pH.)

The patient is placed in the supine position. PKP is performed under general or local standby anesthesia, depending on the surgeon's preference. In this description, general anesthesia is used. General anesthesia affords more control for the surgeon against an expulsive hemorrhage in this "open-sky" technique. A Foley catheter is placed into the bladder by the circulating nurse. Intraocular pressure is lowered by 50 cc of 25% Mannitol (Astra USA, Inc., Westboro, MA) administered intravenously. The operative eye is inspected digitally by the surgeon and softness noted. The OA prepares and drapes the patient in sterile fashion. A lid speculum is placed in the eye by the OA or the surgeon. The OA hands a #12 radial blade marker to the surgeon, who marks the center of the cornea with gentian violet. The gentian violet creates a visual radial grid for the

LABORATORY VALUES

Were any of the following laboratory tests performed? ☐ Yes ☐ No If "Yes," complete the following as applies.

Most Recent WBC: __________ Date:___/___/___ Comment:____________________

Abnormal WBC: __________ Date:___/___/___ Comment:____________________

Abnormal WBC: __________ Date:___/___/___ Comment:____________________

Admitting WBC: __________ Date:___/___/___ Comment:____________________

Most Recent Blood Culture: Date:___/___/___ Result: ☐ No Growth Times _____ Days ☐ Positive for Growth

If Positive, Specify Organism(s): ____________________

Other Pertinent Lab Values: ☐ Yes ☐ No____________________

____

____

SEROLOGY

Blood Drawn by: ____________________ Date & Time Drawn:___/___/___ ________ Site:__________

Serum Specimen Archived? ☐ Yes ☐ No Date:___/___/___

☐ Yes ☐ No Elisa Test for HIV-1 & 2 Comb. Antibody Performed? Date:___/___/___ Results: ☐ Reactive ☐ Non-Reactive

☐ Yes ☐ No Hepatitis B Surface Antigen Test Performed? Date:___/___/___ Results: ☐ Reactive ☐ Non-Reactive

☐ Yes ☐ No Hepatitis C Antibody Test Performed? Date:___/___/___ Results: ☐ Reactive ☐ Non-Reactive

☐ Yes ☐ No Syphilis Screening (RPR/VDRL) Performed? Date:___/___/___ Results: ☐ Reactive ☐ Non-Reactive

☐ Yes ☐ No Elisa Test for HTLV-1 Antibody Performed? Date:___/___/___ Results: ☐ Reactive ☐ Non-Reactive

Other Serology: ____________________ Date:___/___/___ Results: ☐ Reactive ☐ Non-Reactive

Other Serology: ____________________ Date:___/___/___ Results: ☐ Reactive ☐ Non-Reactive

Were re-tests performed for reactive screening tests? ☐ Yes ☐ No If "Yes," complete the following.

Test Performed: ____________________ Date:___/___/___ Results: __________

Test Performed: ____________________ Date:___/___/___ Results: __________

Serology Performed by: ____________________

Lab I.D. # 020584

PATHOLOGY

Autopsy Performed? ☐ Yes ☐ No Locator: ____________________ Date:___/___/___

Gross Autopsy Findings:____________________

____________________ Evidence of High Risk Exposure? ☐ Yes ☐ No

Pathologist: ____________________ Findings Reported by: ____________________

Findings Received by: ____________________ Date:___/___/___ Time ________

Figure 10-1. Laboratory values, serology, and pathology report form. (Form provided by The Lions Bank of Delaware Valley, Philadelphia, PA.)

GENERAL INFORMATION

Donor Number: _____

Donor Name: _____ Age: _____ Sex: ☐ Male ☐ Female

Race: ☐ Caucasian ☐ Hispanic ☐ African American ☐ Asian ☐ Native American ☐ Other: _____

Date of Birth: ____/____/____ Social Security Number: _____

Next of Kin: _____ Relation: _____ Phone: _____

Address: _____ City: _____ State: _____ Zip: _____

Letter Sent NOK? ☐ Yes ☐ No

Institution: _____ Unit: _____

City: _____ State: _____ Contacted by: _____

Pronounced by: _____ Patient ID Number: _____

Letter Sent Hospital? ☐ Yes ☐ No

Referral by: _____ Time: _____

Attending Physician(s): _____ Phone: _____

Organ Donor? ☐ Yes ☐ No   Other Tissue Donor? ☐ Yes ☐ No   Recorded Consent on File: ☐ Yes ☐ No

Medical Examiner Case? ☐ Yes ☐ No Released by: _____

Case Number: _____ Location: _____

Date of Admission:	____/____/____ Time: _____	Total Time of Body Refrigeration:	_____ Hours
Date of Expiration:	____/____/____ Time: _____	Expiration to Enucleation Time Interval:	_____ Hours
Declared Brain Dead:	____/____/____ Time: _____	Expiration to Preservation Time Interval:	_____ Hours
Date of Enucleation/In Situ:	____/____/____ Time: _____	Enucleation/In Situ Performed by: _____	
Date of Preservation:	____/____/____ Time: _____	Preservation Performed by: _____	

LIONS EYE BANK OF DELAWARE VALLEY
Wills Eye Hospital
900 Walnut Street
Philadelphia, PA 19107
800-462-1011 • 215-627-0700
Charter Member — Eye Bank Association of America

MEDICAL HISTORY

Cause of Death: _____

Admitting Diagnosis: _____

Recent History: _____
_____
_____
_____
_____
_____

Figure 10-2. General information and medical history report form. (Form provided by The Lions Bank of Delaware Valley, Philadelphia, PA.)

MEDICAL HISTORY (Cont.)

Past History: ☐ Yes ☐ No _____

_____

_____

Surgeries: ☐ Yes ☐ No _____

_____

Medications: ☐ Yes ☐ No _____

_____

☐ Yes ☐ No   Diabetes, Type: _____ How long? _____

☐ Yes ☐ No   Dialysis Treatments, Specify: _____

☐ Yes ☐ No   Steroid Therapy, Specify: _____

☐ Yes ☐ No   Ventilator Dependence, How Long? _____

☐ Yes ☐ No   Chemotherapy, Specify: _____

☐ Yes ☐ No   Radiation Therapy, Specify: _____

☐ Yes ☐ No   Abnormal Body Temperature, Specify: _____

☐ Yes ☐ No   Jaundice, Specify: _____

☐ Yes ☐ No   Blood Transfusions   (If yes – see back page)

Based on available medical history, do any of the following conditions apply? ☐ Yes ☐ No   If "Yes," indicate below.

☐ Death of Unknown Cause
☐ Central Nervous System Diseases of Unknown Etiology
☐ Creutzfeldt-Jacob Disease
☐ Subacute Sclerosing Panencephalopathy
☐ Progressive Multifocal Leukoencephalopathy
☐ Congenital Rubella
☐ Reyes Syndrome
☐ Active Viral Encephalitis of Unknown Origin
☐ Active Septicemia – Bacteremia, Fungemia, Viremia
☐ Active Bacterial or Fungal Endocarditis
☐ Active Viral Hepatitis
☐ Rabies

☐ Prior Intraocular or Anterior Segment Surgery
☐ Active Leukemias
☐ Active Disseminated Lymphomas
☐ Hepatitis B Surface Antigen Positive
☐ Pil hGH Recipient (1963–1985)
☐ HIV Seropositive or High Risk
☐ Acquired Immunodeficiency Syndrome
☐ Children (<13 yrs.) of Mothers with AIDS or High Risk
☐ HTLV-I or HTLV-II Infection
☐ Active Syphilis
☐ Hepatitis C Seropositive

Based on available medical history, do any of the following conditions apply? ☐ Yes ☐ No   If "Yes," indicate below.

☐ Retinoblastoma
☐ Malignant Tumors of the Eye
☐ Active Ocular or Intraocular Inflammation
☐ Glaucoma

☐ Corneal Disease
☐ Ocular Surgery
☐ Trauma

BODY TEMPERATURE CONVERSION TABLE

FAHRENHEIT	CELSIUS	FAHRENHEIT	CELSIUS
96.8	36.0	102.0	39.0
97.7	36.5	103.2	39.5
98.6	37.0	104.0	40.0
99.5	37.5	104.9	40.5
100.4	38.0	105.8	41.0
101.3	38.5		

Figure 10-3. Medical history report form. (Form provided by The Lions Bank of Delaware Valley, Philadelphia, PA.)

MEDICAL/ SOCIAL HISTORY

Information Documented by:_____   Date: _____ /_____ /_____   Time: _____

Source of Information:_____   Relationship to Deceased: _____

Do you feel you know the deceased well enough to answer questions regarding the medical/social history?   YES   or   NO

	YES	NO	
1. Ever refused as a blood donor or told not to donate? WHY?			
2. Ever received an organ or tissue transplant? i.e. kidney, heart, bone, cornea, skin, sclera, etc.			
3. Any known history of.			
Heart Disease: HTN, CHF, CAD, Valve Disease, MI, Cardiomyopathy, etc.			
Lung Disease: TB, COPD, Valley Fever, Pneumonia, etc			
Liver Disease: Cirrhosis, Jaundice, Hepatitis (type), etc			
Kidney Disease: Renal Failure, Dialysis, Diabetes, etc			
4. In the past 12 months any vaccinations or immunizations?			
5. Ever vaccinated for Hepatitis-B?			
6. Any change in mental status or neurological disorders? Ex: Memory Loss, Confusion, Dementia, Seizures, MS, CVA or Diagnosis of Alzheimer's, etc.			
7. Any history of Cancer or Blood Disorders?			
Malignancies: Cancers, Metastasis, Leukemia, Chemotherapy, or Radiation, Tx. (types and date of Tx. last Tx received)			
Blood Disorders. Hematological Malignancies, Lymphoma, Multiple Myeloma, etc			
Skin Disorders: Burns, Lesions, Skin Cancers, Kaposi's Sarcoma, etc			
History of Hemophilia? Ever received Human-Derived Clotting Factor?			
8. Any history of Bone/Joint/Connective Tissue Disorders or Autoimmune Disease? Ex. Stiff or Sore Joints, Gout, Osteoporosis, DJD, Systemic Lupus, Arthritis (type)			
9. Any current history of infections or Septicemia? Ex: Sepsis, (viral, bacterial, fungal), Malaria, Endocarditis, etc.			
10. Any history of eye disease or surgery? Ex: Glaucoma, Retinitis Pigmentosa, Retinoblastoma, Prior Surgeries. Laser Surgery for elimination of eye glasses, etc.			
11. Is patient diabetic? (type, length of duration, medications)			
12. Animal Bites/Rabies. Type of Animal (Domestic vs. Wild). Was the animal quarantined? Treatment received by patient.			
13. Toxic Exposures. Lead, Mercury, Gold Fluoride occupational substances. Pesticides, Agent Orange, Asbestos, etc			
14. Any history of hospitalization within the last 2 years (dates, treatment rendered)?			
Medications: Current Medications, Steroid Tx., etc. Surgeries. What type?			
Ever receive Human Pituitary Growth Hormone?			
15. Social History:			
a. Tobacco Usage - Amount			
b. ETOH Usage - Amount			
c. Tattoos - Date			
d. Any Body Piercing, Acupuncture or Accidental needle stick in the past year? When? Where?			
e. Travel outside the USA in the past year? When? Where?			
f. Ever been incarcerated (in prison)? When? Where?			
g. Ever lived in a long term psychiatric or MR facility? When? Where?			
h. Ever used self-injected street drugs? When? Where?			
i. Ever use street drugs? Ex: Cocaine, Marijuana, Crack, etc.			

Figure 10-4. Medical/social history and physical inspection form. (Form provided by The Lions Bank of Delaware Valley, Philadelphia, PA.)

MEDICAL/ SOCIAL HISTORY

Medical/Social History Continued →

	YES	NO	
16. Diagnosis of AIDS or any of the following: Unexplained Weight Loss, Night Sweats, Blue or Purple Spots on Skin or Mucous Membranes, Enlarged Lymph Nodes, Fever greater than 100.5 F for over 10 Days, Persistent Cough, SOB, Recurrent Infections, Unexplained Persistent Diarrhea.			
17. Diagnosis or signs of Hepatitis: Jaundice, Enlarged Liver or spleen, Elevated ALT, Unexplained Malaise, Nausea, Pale Stool or Dark Colored Urine.			
18. Any history of direct or sexual contact with IV drug users, male to male sex, male homosexuals, bisexuals, prostitutes, hemophiliacs or any sexually transmitted diseases? Ex. Syphilis, Gonorrhea, etc.			
19. History of, or currently having contact with anyone having or being at risk for AIDS or Hepatitis?			
20. Name of personal physician, ophthalmologist or specialist – phone number.			

PHYSICAL INSPECTION

Gross Body Examination: Indicate lacerations, abrasions, tattoos, IV sites, airways, melanomas, ulcers or other identifying marks. Write the word **none** if there are no marks present.

Neck: _____   Groin: _____
Chest: _____   Abdomen: _____
Head: _____   Left Leg: _____
Left Arm: _____   Left Foot: _____
Left Hand: _____   Right Leg: _____
Right Arm: _____   Right Foot: _____
Right Hand: _____   Back: _____

Indications of IV Drug Abuse: Yes No Specify: _____

General Impression of Donor's Appearance: _____   Height: _____   Weight: _____

Pre-recovery Gross Penlight Examination of Corneal-Scleral Segment

Is cornea clear?	YES	NO	Is the epithelium intact?	YES	NO
Are any foreign objects present?	YES`	NO	Is preservation medium clear?	YES	NO
Scleral Color?_____			Circle: Aphakic Phakic Pseudophakic		

Problems associated with eye tissue recovery and intervention and interventions taken?_____

I have viewed the facial features after eye enucleation or in situ and observed no discoloration of the eye area.

Signed:_____   Time of Viewing:_____

Please Note any Facial Problems:_____

Figure 10-4 (continued). Medical/social history and physical inspection form. (Form provided by The Lions Bank of Delaware Valley, Philadelphia, PA.)

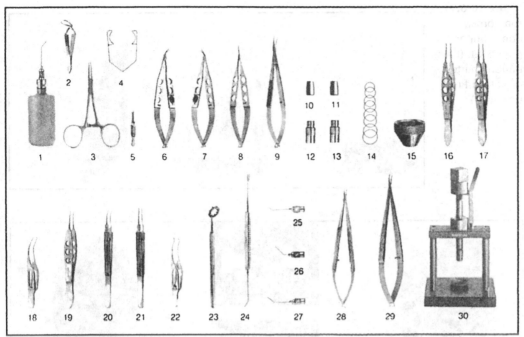

Figure 10-5. Suggested corneal transplant set. (Set illustration courtesy of Katena Products, Inc.)

1. BSS Irrigator
2. Towel Clamp (2)
3. Mosquito Forceps (2)
4. Wire Speculum
5. Serrefine
6. Transplant Scissors, left
7. Transplant Scissors, right
8. Vannas Scissors
9. Stitch Scissors
10. Trephine Blade, 7.5 mm
11. Trephine Blade, 8.0 mm
12. Trephine Handle, 7.5 mm
13. Trephine Handle, 8.0 mm
14. Fixation Ring Set
15. Intraoperative Keratometer
16. Superior Rectus Forceps
17. Fixation Forceps, 0.3 mm
18. Colibri Forceps, 0.12 mm
19. Corneal Forceps, 0.12 mm
20. Tying Forceps, curved
21. Tying Forceps, straight
22. Double Corneal Fixation Forceps
23. Suture Placement Marker
24. Paton Spatula
25. Air Injection Cannula, 30 gauge
26. Viscoelastic Injection Cannula, 26 gauge
27. Viscoelastic Aspiration Cannula, 22 gauge
28. Needle Holder, micro
29. Needle Holder, standard
30. Donor Button Punch

surgeon to use in preparing to trephine (cut) the host cornea. The donor tissue is then removed from the OptiSol medium and passed to the surgeon. The donor tissue is placed on a Teflon (E.I. DuPont Company, Wilmington, DE) punch block, epithelial side down so that cell loss will not be incurred. A corneal trephine is selected by the surgeon, usually 0.2 to 0.5 mm larger as determined by the recipient measurement. The trephine is used to punch the donor tissue from the endothelial side (Figure 10-6). Care is taken by the OA to cover any exposed trephine blades. The OA places the residual donor tissue rim and storage medium in thyroglycolate preservative solution; it is sent to microbiology for culture and sensitivity (C & S). The OA places a few drops of the storage medium to cover the donor button, which is saved for later use. Care is also taken that no bright, drying overhead operating lights are shining on the donor button.

A typical rim is about 2 mm in width, but it may be wider or narrower to encompass or avoid vessels or other pathology. The narrower the rim, the more likely that postoperative vessel

Figure 10-6. Barron corneal donor button punch set. (Illustration courtesy of Katena Products, Inc.)

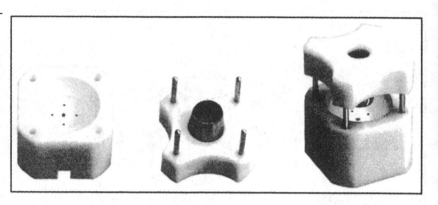

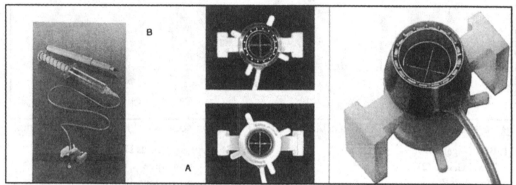

Figure 10-7. A. Barron radial vacuum trephine. B. Trephine sterile set with marking pen. (Illustration courtesy of Katena Products, Inc.)

ingrowth to the sutures, premature suture loosening, peripheral anterior synechiae, glaucoma, and graft rejection may occur. Conversely, the larger the donor graft, the better the postoperative corneal optical performance, the faster the recovery and the less chance that irregular astigmatism will develop.

Attention is now given to the recipient eye. A suction trephination system such as the Hanna or Barron is assembled (Figure 10-7). The area of trephination is marked, suction applied by the assisting surgeon or OA to engage the globe, and the surgeon applies the trephine to a 90% corneal depth. After this is achieved, the suction is released by the OA or assisting surgeon. The OA hands a supersharp blade to the surgeon. The anterior chamber is entered with this blade at the 9 o'clock position. The OA passes the corneal scissors to be used in excising the diseased host tissue. This tissue is removed, placed in a preservative solution, and submitted to pathology. The OA passes curved Vannas scissors to the surgeon to trim the rim of Descemet's membrane. The OA draws up Miochol with a 25G needle on a 3 cc syringe. It is handed to the surgeon to effect miosis of the pupil. A viscoelastic agent is prepared by the OA. The OA hands the surgeon this viscoelastic agent and it is injected into the angle, 360 degrees around, and over the iris plane to reduce trauma to the donor endothelium. The viscoelastic agent is not irrigated from the eye. The donor button is brought over the surgical field and irrigated with a few drops of BSS (balanced salt solution) by the surgeon. The OA prepares a #10-0 nylon suture on a microscopic needle-holder and passes this to the surgeon. The donor button is sutured into place with eight interrupted sutures and a 16-bite running suture. The combination of interrupted and running suture techniques vary according to case specifics. The suture knots are buried in the recipient tissue so as not to be exposed. The eye is reformed with BSS. The wound is inspected by the surgeon and found to be water tight. The OA opens a fluorescein strip. This is passed to the surgeon who applies it to the surface of the graft to assess any shallow placement of running suture, prior to patching. A suture that is too tight would create a "doughnut effect" of the donor graft. At this point, the surgeon would adjust the suture accordingly.

The OA draws up cefazolin, gentamicin, and dexamethasone into 3 cc syringes with 25G needles. These are injected subconjunctivally by the surgeon. The OA hands the surgeon a collagen protective corneal shield which is soaked in equal parts of steroidal, anti-inflammatory, and antibiotic solution (5 drops of each) for 10 minutes prior. This shield is left on the new cornea for a period of 24 hours. The eye is coated with a viscoelastic agent followed by an antibiotic ointment, a patch, and an eye shield.

Pterygium

A pterygium is a wing-shaped, benign, conjunctival growth over the cornea, usually originating from the inner canthal aspect of the eye. This tissue crosses the limbus and adheres to Bowman's membrane. Superficial layers of the stroma and Bowman's membrane are destroyed as a result. Pterygia are almost always preceded and accompanied by pingueculae, a degenerative lesion of the bulbar conjunctiva occurring as a result of a chemical change in the tissue from radiant UV light exposure. A pterygium does not adhere to the sclera. When a pterygium grows and encroaches on the visual axis of the cornea, surgical removal may be indicated.

Environmental factors such as wind and sun are thought to cause this condition. The most severe occurrences and recurrences are found in warm climates. Genetic predisposition may also be an important factor.

Frequent occurrence of inflammation and infection, restriction of ocular motility, progressive astigmatism, and undesirable cosmetic appearance are all factors that may be considered in removal of the growth.

To keep the cornea clear and guard against recurrence of the pterygium, promising new surgical techniques are being explored with the use of a conjunctival autograft. A graft of conjunctival tissue from the patient is sutured in place after removal of the pterygium. This procedure has been successful against further regrowth. Traditional methods using postoperative beta radiation to the bare sclera, without the use of a graft, have not completely eradicated the incidence of regrowth.

Operative Procedure: Excision of Pterygium with Conjunctival Autograft

After appropriate sterile gown and gloving, the scrub OA drapes the mayo stand in sterile fashion and organizes the instrument tray.

After placing the patient in the supine position, the operative eye (identified by either the OA or the attending surgeon) is prepared and draped in the appropriate sterile fashion. Local anesthesia is administered with additional anesthesia on stand-by. Lidocaine 4% and tetracaine 0.5% are applied topically to the corneal surface by the OA. Lidocaine 4% is placed in the superior and inferior cul-de-sac to provide continuous topical anesthesia. The OA hands the lid speculum to the surgeon and it is placed into the eye. A 3 cc syringe of lidocaine 1% with epinephrine is prepared with a 25G needle and handed to the surgeon for injection into the subconjunctival space nasally and superiorly. The OA passes a #69 crescent-shaped knife to the surgeon, who removes a 4 mm x 4 mm area of conjunctiva and pterygium. The corneal limbus is scraped. The OA prepares the excised specimen for pathology by placing it in a labeled sterile container filled with a storage medium such as formaldehyde. The OA gives the surgeon a disposable hi-temp cautery, which is used to cauterize the scleral base. A fresh 4 mm x 4 mm conjunctival patch is excised superiorly and placed onto the bare scleral area. The OA prepares a #9-0 Vicryl suture on the microscopic needle holder. This is passed to the surgeon, and the conjunctival graft is sutured in place using several interrupted sutures. The lid speculum is removed by either the OA or the surgeon. The pledget of lidocaine 4% is removed by the OA. The OA applies dexamethasone ointment and a pressure patch.

Chapter 11

Refractive Surgery

- As in all elective procedures, the patient's expectations must be consistent with the range of probable outcomes.

- Patients having refractive surgery need to be aware that the goal of the procedure is to reduce their dependency on glasses or contact lenses.

- Those who insist on having perfect vision at all times are not good candidates for refractive surgery.

- Refractive procedures are often performed in fractions of a micron; therefore, preoperative testing must be accurate in order to allow the technology to fully realize its potential.

- In preparing the surgical instruments and lasers used in refractive surgery, the OA is responsible for the meticulous cleaning, sterilization, and calibration of the equipment.

- Intraoperatively during incisional techniques, the role of the OA is to act as a scrub nurse. In laser techniques, particularly in lamellar keratoplasty, the OA is responsible for laser calibration and patient comfort.

Introduction and History of Refractive Surgery

Refractive surgery consists of changing the refractive status of the eye to reduce or eliminate myopia, astigmatism, and hyperopia. For the purpose of this chapter, we will confine the discussion to the corneal restructuring procedures of radial and astigmatic keratotomy (RK and AK), photorefractive keratectomy (PRK), and laser in situ keratomileusis (LASIK).

In 1960, Russian ophthalmologist Svyatoslav Fyodorov performed RK using anterior keratotomy. Leo Bores introduced RK to the United States in 1978. In the early 1990s, Charles Casebeer created a systematic approach to RK and its enhancements via consistent instructional courses. The 10 year Prospective Evaluation of Radial Keratotomy (PERK) study demonstrated excellent safety and efficacy of refractive procedures, but less predictability. With the evolution of excimer laser technology, the role of RK has now been markedly reduced to primarily the treatment of lower levels of myopia.

Excimer laser technology for ophthalmic purposes began clinical use in the 1980s. After exhaustive studies, PRK was approved in the United States in 1995. PRK was not effective in the 1980's for the treatment of high myopia. Another laser refractive procedure known as LASIK has emerged, combining the advantages of PRK and keratomileusis.[1]

Radial Keratotomy and Astigmatic Keratotomy

RK is an incisional corneal keratotomy procedure that utilizes radial incisions placed in the peripheral 2/3 of the cornea at approximately 95% corneal depth, sparing a central optical zone. Its purpose is to flatten the central cornea. The number of incisions and the diameter of the central zone is determined by the patient's myopic refraction and age. AK is the placement of arctype incisions (in the mid-periphery) of various lengths and distances from the central cornea that flatten the steep axis on which they are placed. The length and distance from the corneal center are determined by the patient's astigmatic error and age.

RK/AK Patient and Equipment Preparation

The OA is responsible for proper setup of surgical instruments (Figure 11-1), and in some practices, the calibration, setting, and confirmation of the keratome setting. The OA positions the patient comfortably on the OR bed or chair, and aligns the eye with the OR microscope. Once the patient is comfortable and the scope is properly adjusted, the OA preps and drapes the patient in the usual manner. Although it is ultimately the surgeon's responsibility, it is helpful for the OA to inspect the eyelids and adnexa for any sign of infection prior to surgery. The OA should also inquire if the patient has had any recent illness since last seeing the physician.

Operative Procedure: Combined RK/AK

The patient is brought to the procedure room by the OA and prepped and draped in the usual manner. The speculum is handed to the surgeon by the OA. Pachymetry is obtained temporal to the pupil. The OA announces the pachymetry setting to the surgeon. Diamond micrometer blades are set to 100% of the pachymetry reading (varies per surgeon). The surgeon asks for the appropriate optical zone (OZ) marker. The surgeon then asks for the arc markers from the OA; the markers are used to indicate one or two AK incisions on the steep axis. The OA receives the arc

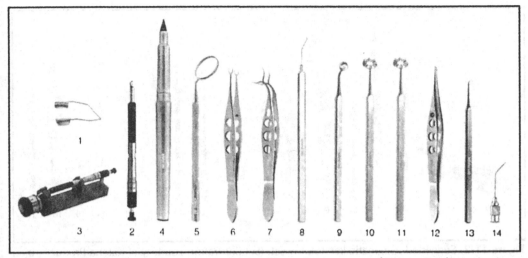

Figure 11-1. Suggested radial keratotomy set. (Set illustration courtesy of Katena Products, Inc.)

1. Wire Speculum, solid
2. Diamond Micrometer, double edge
3. Blade Gauge
4. Marking Pen
5. Thornton Fixing Ring
6. Fixation Forceps, straight
7. Fixation Forceps, angled

8. Visual Axis Marker
9. Optic Zone Marker
10. Radial Marker, 6 lines
11. Radial Marker, 8 lines
12. Incision Spreading Forceps
13. Incision Depth Gauge
14. Irrigating Cannula, 27 gauge

marker and hands the surgeon the radial marker so that the appropriate number of incisions can be marked. All incisions are to 95% depth. On conclusion of the case, an anti-inflammatory, non-steroidal, and antibiotic are placed in the operative eye by the OA. The OA instructs the patient on postoperative care and schedules follow-up in the office in one day.

PRK

PRK is the application of ultraviolet energy at 193 mm which vaporizes anterior corneal tissue by breaking molecular bonds. Each laser burst results in corneal thinning of approximately 1/4 of a micron. By varying the depth of ablation and diameter of the ablated zone, various amounts of myopia can be corrected. Energy can be delivered in astigmatic patterns to correct myopia and astigmatism simultaneously (Figure 11-2).

Typical PRK Surgical Tray

Leiberman speculum
Fukasaku hockey knife
Paton spatula

Katena fixation ring
Optic zone marker, 7 mm
McPherson tying forceps

PRK Patient and Equipment Preparation

Prior to bringing the patient to the excimer suite, the laser is calibrated and tested by the OA following the manufacturers' instructions. Some machines prevent the operator from proceeding should any fault be found. However, in the event that any flaw is detected in the calibration pro-

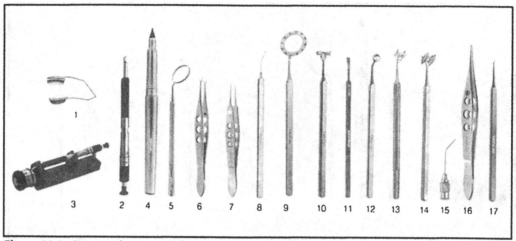

Figure 11-2. Suggested astigmatic keratotomy set. (Set illustration courtesy of Katena Products, Inc.)

1. Wire Speculum, solid
2. Diamond Micrometer, double edge
3. Blade Gauge
4. Marking Pen
5. Thornton Fixing Ring
6. Fixation Forceps, double
7. Fixation Forceps, 0.12 mm
8. Visual Axis Marker
9. Degree Gauge
10. Axis Marker
11. T-Incision Marker
12. Optic Zone Marker
13. Thornton Corneal Marker
14. Arcuate Incision marker
15. Irrigating Cannula, 27 gauge
16. Incision Spreading Forceps
17. Incision Depth Gauge

cedure or test mode, the case must be canceled until the machine is operating perfectly. Once the laser is ready for surgery, the patient's desired correction is entered. The patient is then brought to the operating room and positioned by the OA at the laser. Anesthetic eye drops are placed in each eye and the opposite eye is taped closed for the purpose of fixation. The patient is then positioned underneath the laser microscope and the surgery proceeds (after the OA and surgeon confirm the desired correction and the proper working order of the laser).

Operative Procedure: PRK

The patient is brought to the laser suite and prepped in the usual manner by the OA. The first eye is centered under the microscope and the OA hands the surgeon a 7 mm corneal marker (previously coated with a blue marking pen by the OA). The surgeon marks the central cornea with a firm placement of the marker, and is given the Touck knife by the OA. The epithelium is debrided. The OA hands a surgical spear to the surgeon's other hand to allow for stabilization of the eye. The epithelium is removed from the perimeter towards the center and placed onto the surgical spear. The OA hands the surgeon a dry surgical spear to sweep the debrided area, and then another spear mildly soaked in carboxymethylcellulose sodium 1% lubricant to coat the exposed area lightly in order to smooth the surface. The surgeon then confirms with the OA that the laser is ready to be activated and the procedure begins. The OA announces how much time is left in the procedure in 10 second increments so that the surgeon will continuously encourage the patient to remain fixated on the aiming beam. Upon conclusion of the case, the OA hands the surgeon a bandage contact lens using either a forceps or surgical spear. Antibiotic and/or steroidal eye drops are placed into the operative eye by the OA. In the event that the second eye is done at the same sitting, the first eye is taped shut by the OA and the desired correction for the second eye is entered

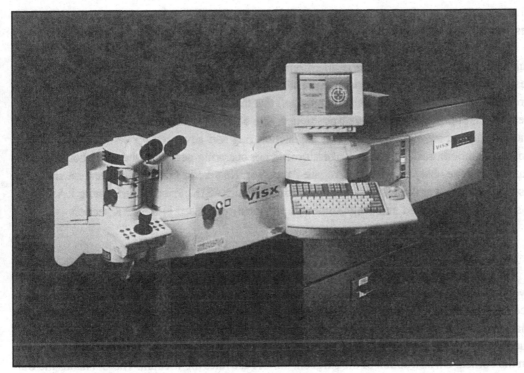

Figure 11-3. VISX excimer laser. (Photo courtesy of VISX.)

in the laser. The machine is now recalibrated by the OA while the surgeon places the microscope over the second eye. The OA places an anesthetic drop in the second eye. Upon conclusion of the second eye, the OA helps the patient from the operating table and accompanies him to the slit lamp. A slit lamp exam will ensure proper placement of the bandage contact lens as well as the integrity of the procedure.

LASIK Defined

LASIK utilizes a microkeratome to create a 160 degree micron flap. The flap is flipped to the side on its "hinge" to expose a stromal bed, which is then treated with excimer laser. (Figure 11-3) The hinge is then redeposited and self-sticks without sutures. Visual recovery is expected in 1 to 4 days. Typically, medications are discontinued in less than 1 week. The rapid recovery, decreased pain, and reduction of corneal haze gives LASIK significant advantages over PRK, particularly in higher amounts of astigmatism.

Typical LASIK Surgical Tray

Lieberman speculum	Marking pen
Corneal marker	Microkeratome instrumentation
Spatula	McPherson tying forceps

LASIK Patient and Instrumentation Preparation

Ninety percent of the LASIK procedure is the creation of the flap by the microkeratome. A well-performed flap procedure requires adequate lid exposure and a debris-free area. The OA should clean and irrigate the fornices preoperatively. The OA then places topical anesthesia and antibiotic drops in the operative eye prior to the procedure. Following ablation, debris may float and remain between the flap and stromal bed. Irrigation, which may be done by the OA with BSS, lessens the risk of infection.

Care and preparation of the microkeratome instrument is the most important step in successful LASIK. The microkeratome is an extremely delicate instrument, and the slightest flaw can result in aborted cases or disappointing results. The OA must be sure that the gears are working properly in a forward and reverse direction and that the 160 micron plate used to define the thickness of the flap is in place and well-positioned. The blade is examined under the microscope, and the microkeratome must be placed in the suction ring and advanced forward and backward to ensure a smooth track. If the microkeratome is not operating perfectly, the case should not and cannot be done. Only Palmolive (Colgate-Palmolive, New York, NY) liquid detergent should be used when cleaning the instrumentation involved with LASIK. Prior to performing LASIK, the laser must be calibrated and programmed as previously discussed in the PRK section.

Operative Procedure: LASIK

The OA preps and drapes the eye in the usual manner, making sure that the drape covers the eyelid margins. Adequate exposure is obtained, and the eye is centered underneath the microscope. The alignment markers (which have previously been coated with a marking pen) are placed in the periphery of the cornea by the surgeon. The OA hands the surgeon the pneumatic suction ring in the hand opposite of the operative eye. The ring is seated firmly and slightly nasal on the cornea. On instruction of the surgeon, the OA activates the vacuum. The OA hands the Barraquer tonometer to the surgeon who, after checking intraocular pressure, hands it immediately back to the OA. While the pressure is being checked, the OA picks up the microkeratome with the other hand. The microkeratome is now handed overhand to the surgeon (same hand as the operative eye). The microkeratome is inserted into the tracts and advanced fully by the surgeon. At this point the surgical field is inspected by the surgeon and the OA. If there are any obstacles such as lashes, excess lid tissue, chemotic conjunctiva, or foreign bodies, the OA must assist the surgeon in holding back or removing the obstacles. Only then can the surgeon proceed to depress the forward pedal until the hinge stop is reached. Prior to advancing the keratome, the OA moistens the corneal bed with BSS. The surgeon then pushes the reverse pedal and, as soon as the microkeratome is fully retreated, immediately tells the OA to remove suction. The OA takes the microkeratome apparatus from the surgeon and exchanges it for a cyclodialysis-type spatula, which the surgeon uses to retract the flap and expose the stromal bed. The bed is then ablated. The OA hands the surgeon a syringe of filtered BSS with a small gauge cannula which is used to reposition and irrigate beneath the flap (to clean interface foreign bodies). Using a surgical spear, the flap is aligned. Drying along the edge occurs, encouraging flap adhesion. After 2 to 3 minutes the peripheral cornea is depressed with a dry surgical spear in an attempt to identify striae in the adhesed flap. An antibiotic and steroid medication is applied. The eye is then taped shut if the second eye is going to be done immediately. On conclusion of the second procedure, the flap location is confirmed with a slit lamp before the patient leaves the OR suite.

Intraoperative Complications of LASIK: The OA's Role

LASIK procedures are unique in their flap complications:

- Lamellar incision may be too short (pupil bisection). If the OA notices that the flap is too short, he or she must notify the surgeon immediately. In these cases the procedure should be aborted and rescheduled in approximately 3 months (when the cornea has healed).

- Lamellar incision maybe too long (free cap). The OA should have an antidesiccation chamber available. The free corneal cap should be placed epithelial surface down on a drop of BSS to help preserve the epithelium.

- Lamellar incision of poor quality that is superficial in thickness could result in an irregular, thin, or perforated flap. When an irregular bed is noticed, the case should be aborted and re-attempted in approximately 3 months. The OA needs to clean, sterilize, and check all equipment (including the blade) prior to another case. Thin or perforated corneal flaps occur because of poor blade quality and sharpness, inadequate suction pressure, and/or microkeratome malfunction.

- Corneal perforation or amputation is the most serious complication in LASIK. Corneal perforation and amputation can result in expulsion of ocular contents. The OA and the surgeon must follow a preoperative check list which includes checking the plate in the microkeratome. To avoid any complications intraoperatively, the entire staff, including surgeon, OA, and circulator, must be completely trained and educated in LASIK procedure and management.[1]

Reference

1. Machat JM. *Excimer Laser Refractive Surgery—Practice and Principles*. Thorofare, NJ: SLACK Incorporated; 1996.

Glaucoma

- Candidates for glaucoma surgery often have a higher level of anxiety, as they live with the threat of blindness. For them, conservative medical treatment has failed to arrest the progress of their disease and surgical or laser treatment becomes a necessity.

- Preoperatively, the glaucoma patient should understand that filtering surgery is only the initial part of the management of glaucoma. Postoperative management is critical to the success of the operation.

- Knowledgeable and skillful assistance during manipulation of the conjunctiva and delicate scleral flap is critical to the success of glaucoma surgery.

- The use of antimetabolites and chemotherapeutic agents necessitate careful adherence to protocol by the OA in the handling and disposal of these toxic substances during the surgical procedure.

Glaucoma Defined

The disease process known as glaucoma is the result of increased intraocular pressure (IOP) within the eye. Permanent visual loss results from destructive pressure on the optic disc when elevated pressure is left untreated. As the entire optic nerve is damaged, progressive constriction of the visual field occurs over a long period of time; blindness results.

Contrary to what patients may think, IOP has no direct correlation to blood pressure. It is similar to hypertension in that it is not subjectively felt by the patient when elevated. Like high blood pressure, glaucoma is controlled, not cured.

Glaucoma Classifications and Surgical Procedures

Open-Angle Glaucoma

Chronic open-angle glaucoma (COAG) is the result of sustained IOP increase due to inadequate aqueous humor drainage, manifesting in optic nerve damage. Vision is destroyed gradually and painlessly in COAG. The sieve-like drainage structure known as the trabecular meshwork (TM) is often treated with the argon laser in a procedure known as argon laser trabeculoplasty (ALT). ALT creates new channels within the TM to facilitate drainage of the fluid. With the aid of a mirrored gonioscopic lens, laser burns are placed at equal intervals in the TM.

Trabeculectomy is a fistulizing procedure where a small portion of the TM is surgically removed through a scleral flap, allowing the aqueous humor to flow out of the anterior chamber. The aqueous humor pools in a pocket or bleb under the conjunctiva.

Filtration surgery can fail secondary to an accelerated healing response. This results in conjunctival scarring and eventual closure of the filtration site. Eyes considered to be at high risk for the failure of filtering surgery include those with active inflammation of the anterior segment (as in iritis), neovascular glaucoma, or proliferative diabetic retinopathy. Young patients are also at risk, as well as those who have had previous surgery to that eye or in whom the fellow eye has undergone filtering surgery that failed because of rapid healing. Antimetabolites are chemotherapeutic agents which prevent the production of new collagen that results in scar tissue. When introduced as part of the filtration procedure, these substances better control and minimize the healing response. In high-risk situations, 5-Fluorouracil (5-FU), injected subconjunctivally, has shown to be an effective antimetabolite. Mitomycin C (a more potent antimetabolite than 5-FU) is applied intraoperatively, avoiding postoperative subconjunctival injections. Mitomycin C has proven extremely useful in the management of glaucoma in children, in whom postoperative injections are difficult.

Tube/shunt procedures using implants such as the Molteno, Baerveldt, and Krupin, are an important treatment option in the management of very complicated glaucoma, especially cases that do not respond well to conventional filtering surgery. In these procedures, a small-caliber silicone tube is introduced into either the anterior chamber or (in the case of a postvitrectomy eye) the posterior chamber. The tube drains to an external reservoir system that maintains an area of filtration, often quite far back on the globe. Filtration occurs through the surface of the capsule that develops over the reservoir. The Krupin valve implant, which is the operative procedure described in this chapter, is designed to avoid excessive hypotony (excessively low IOP) of the eye after surgery.

Cyclodestructive procedures are those that destroy the ciliary body to achieve a decrease in aqueous humor production. Cycloablation is usually reserved for eyes considered to be poor surgical candidates, and is usually performed under retrobulbar anesthesia. The ciliary body can be treated via endoscopic laser photocoagulation. Laser cyclophotocoagulation (CPC) is a cyclodestructive procedure that is rapidly replacing cyclocryotherapy (where a freezing probe is applied externally on the globe to destroy the ciliary body).

Angle-Closure Glaucoma

Complete blockage of the drainage system is known as angle-closure glaucoma (ACG). Nd:YAG laser is the treatment most often selected where the surgeon creates a laser peripheral iridotomy (LPI) to relieve the pressure. In most cases, Nd:YAG iridotomy is preferred as a simpler and faster technique than argon laser iridotomy. It is of importance to note that all laser procedures can result in a transient rise in IOP which must be carefully monitored postoperatively. The use of aproclonidine 0.5% perioperatively is often implemented to prevent these pressure spikes. A surgical peripheral iridectomy (PI) may be done later if the iridotomy does not remain open.

Operative Procedure: Trabeculectomy with Intraoperative Mitomycin C

The patient is brought to the OR and placed in the supine position. IV sedation is administered by the attending anesthetist. Local retrobulbar or peribulbar anesthesia is applied to the operative eye using a combination of lidocaine, Marcaine, and Wydase. Digital pressure is briefly maintained on the globe by the surgeon to distribute the anesthetic effect. The eye is then prepped and draped in the usual sterile fashion.

A lid speculum is passed to the surgeon for appropriate positioning. (Figure 12-1) The OA prepares either an #8-0 Vicryl on a spatulated needle or #6-0 silk suture (surgeon's preference) on the needleholder. This is given to the surgeon who then passes it twice through the cornea as a stay suture. Next, the eye is rotated inferiorly via the stay suture which is attached inferiorly to the surgical drape with a 1/4 inch sterile strip or hemostat. In the limbal-based approach, Westcott scissors are passed to the surgeon by the OA where they are used to make a circumferential conjunctival incision approximately 10 mm posterior to the surgical limbus in the superior quadrant. Again, depending on the approach, either fornix-based or limbal-based flaps are made. In either case, careful tissue manipulation with nontoothed forceps by the OA is critical to prevent any perforations or "button-holing" of the fragile conjunctival tissue. This incision is carried down to bare sclera and extended both nasally and temporally for approximately 10 mm in total length. Both sharp and blunt dissection with the Westcott scissors is then used to carry the conjunctiva and Tenon's tissue down onto the anterior cornea. The OA attaches the bipolar forceps to the Wetfield cautery and passes them to the surgeon for hemostasis. The OA places a #57 blade in the blade handle or opens a single-use crescent-shaped blade and passes this to the surgeon. This blade is then used to outline a 4 x 4 mm, half scleral thickness flap with a 4 mm limbal base. Next, a drainage sponge soaked in Mitomycin C (0.2 to 0.5 mg per cc) is placed on top of the outlined scleral flap by the surgeon with conjunctiva and Tenon's tissue draped over it. This drain placement is often performed with single-use forceps for complete disposal of this toxic substance. The OA notes the time of the placement and after 3 minutes the sponge is removed by the surgeon and

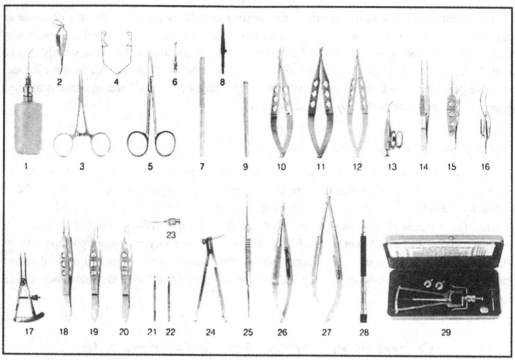

Figure 12-1. Suggested glaucoma surgery set. (Set illustration courtesy of Katena Products, Inc.)

1. BSS Irrigator
2. Towel Clamp (2)
3. Mosquito Forceps (2)
4. Wire Speculum
5. Utility Forceps
6. Sclerotome Blade
7. Blade Handle
8. Super Sharp Blade
9. Blade Handle
10. Westcott Scissors
11. Stitch Scissors
12. Vannas Scissors
13. Iris Scissors
14. Dressing Forceps
15. Bishop-Harmon Forceps
16. Colibri Forceps, 0.12 mm
17. Caliper
18. Suturing Forceps, 0.12 mm
19. Tying Forceps, straight
20. Tying Forceps, angled
21. Trabeculotomy Probe, right
22. Trabeculotomy Probe, left
23. Air Injection Cannula, 27 gauge
24. Corneoscleral Punch
25. Cyclodialysis Spatula
26. Needle Holder, micro
27. Needle Holder, standard
28. Diamond Step Knife
29. Tonometer

the area is well irrigated with 15 to 30 cc of BSS. It is then dried with an absorbable spear-tipped sponge. Catching all fluids in the plastic drape pocket of the surgical drape and disposing of this chemotherapeutic substance per hospital protocol is very important.

The OA again passes the #57 or crescent blade to the surgeon, who uses it to dissect the scleral flap anteriorly onto clear cornea. A 15° blade is handed to the surgeon by the OA and used to make a paracentesis. The OA then passes a syringe filled with Miostat or Miochol (drugs that induce pupillary constriction) to the surgeon, who injects it through this incision. Next, the super blade is used to enter the anterior chamber along the base of the scleral flap. A Descemet's punch is passed to the surgeon, who excises sclera, creating a sclerostomy. The Vannas scissors are passed to the surgeon by the OA and a peripheral iridectomy is created. During this procedure the OA may be asked to hold the scleral flap. Care must be taken not to evulse or pull the tissue away from the base. Use of the assistant scope by the OA is critical at this juncture. The OA prepares the #10-0 nylon suture on a nonlocking needleholder and passes it to the surgeon. The scleral flap is closed. A 3 cc syringe with an irrigation cannula is filled with BSS by the OA. The surgeon injects this into the anterior chamber through the paracentesis to reform the anterior chamber and to assess adequate filtration through the sides of the scleral bed. The scleral flap is visually inspected by the surgeon for secure placement.

The OA then prepares the #9-0 Vicryl suture and passes this to the surgeon for a double-layer closure of the Tenon's and overlying conjunctival incisions. Additional BSS is placed into the anterior chamber through the paracentesis by the surgeon to assess that the conjunctival closure is watertight and that there is adequate filtration.

The surgeon removes the corneal stay suture. The patient is given a subconjunctival injection of gentamicin and dexamethasone in the inferior fornix, previously prepared by the OA in two separate 3 cc syringes with 25G, 1/2 inch needles. Atropine drops are placed in the eye by the OA to optimize filtration and maintain a deep anterior chamber. Dexamethasone ointment is applied. The lid speculum is removed by the OA or the surgeon and the eye is patched and shielded.

Operative Procedure: Krupin Valve Insertion

The patient is brought to the OR and placed in the supine position. IV sedation is administered by the attending anesthetist. Local retrobulbar or peribulbar anesthesia is applied to the operative eye using lidocaine, Marcaine, and Wydase. The eye is prepped and draped in the usual sterile fashion and a lid speculum is inserted by the surgeon.

The OA prepares a #6-0 silk suture and hands this to the surgeon. The suture is passed twice through the superior cornea to allow the eye to be inferoducted. Westcott scissors are passed to the surgeon by the OA and a peritomy is performed in the superotemporal quadrant, extending both temporally and nasally along the limbus. A subconjunctival dissection utilizing both Westcott and Metzenbaum scissors is then carried up into the superotemporal quadrant. The OA attaches the bipolar forceps to the Wetfield cautery and passes them to the surgeon for hemostasis.

The Krupin implant is inspected by the surgeon, irrigated with BSS, and placed in the superotemporal quadrant of the globe. The OA prepares the #8-0 nylon suture and passes this to the surgeon. The valve is then sutured to the sclera with two interrupted #8-0 nylon sutures. The placement of the valve is approximately 8 mm posterior to the surgical limbus. This placement is checked by the surgeon to insure that the superior and lateral recti muscles are not entrapped.

Next, the surgeon uses a 23G needle to puncture into the anterior chamber at about the 1:30 position. The Krupin valve tube is then cut by the surgeon and threaded through the puncture opening and into the anterior chamber, ensuring a position anterior to the iris without corneal touch.

A diamond knife is prepared by the OA and passed to the surgeon, who uses it to make a temporal paracentesis through the peripheral clear cornea, allowing the anterior chamber to be reformed with BSS when needed. The OA prepares the #10-0 nylon and passes this to the surgeon, who then anchors it to the sclera with two interrupted sutures. The surgeon then cuts a scleral patch graft by hand, approximately 6 mm x 8 mm, and attaches it to the sclera with interrupted #8-0 Vicryl sutures, prepared by the OA, so as to cover the tube. At this point a #9-0 Vicryl suture is prepared and passed to the surgeon. The #6-0 silk corneal stay suture is removed by the surgeon. Conjunctiva and Tenon's tissue is brought in and tacked down to the limbus at the two corners using interrupted and running #9-0 Vicryl sutures.

The patient is given a subconjunctival injection of dexamethasone and gentamicin as well as a topical drop of atropine. The lid speculum is removed by either the surgeon or OA. Dexamethasone ointment is placed in the eye, which is then patched and shielded by the OA.

Complications of Glaucoma Surgery

Postoperative management is critical to the success of any glaucoma filtering procedure.

In the postoperative workup, careful notation of the patients vision, IOP, anterior chamber depth, inflammation, and bleb size (if applicable) is critical. Pain could indicate a precipitous rise in the IOP, or insufficient flow. Decreased vision could be the result of overfiltration, manifesting in a soft eye, flat chamber, or choroidal detachment. In trabeculectomy, the primary postoperative concern to the surgeon is the management of aqueous flow outward through the scleral flap.

The patient is often instructed to shield the operative eye at night to guard against accidental trauma or rubbing. The OA should remind the patient with a bleb that it is not unusual to experience a foreign body or dry eye sensation.

Chapter 13

Cataract

KEY POINTS

- Lens opacification in the presence of functional impairment (lifestyle disruption secondary to visual loss) may indicate the need for cataract surgery and intraocular lens implantation to accomplish visual recovery and restore normal function.

- Cataract removal can be done via intracapsular or extracapsular extraction, or by phacoemulsification.

- A systemized approach with meticulous attention to detail in the preoperative setup, intraoperative support by ensuring optimal visualization for the surgeon on the operative field, and post-operative care and cleaning of equipment and instruments are the main responsibilities of the OA and necessary for consistent results.

Cataract and Intraocular Lens Implantation

A cataract is an opacified lens resulting from age, medication, systemic disease, or trauma. A cataract may also be congenital in nature. When a cataract interferes with visual lifestyle requirements, the patient may elect surgical correction by lens extraction and replacement with an artificial substitute known as an intraocular lens (IOL).

Cataract extraction is accomplished by three traditional methods.

- Intracapsular Cataract Extraction (ICCE)—In this method the entire lens and capsule are removed through a large surgical incision at the corneal limbus with the use of a cryo probe (cold probe). This technique is rarely in use today because postoperative recovery and incisional healing are longer and complications more numerous.

- Extracapsular Cataract Extraction (ECCE)—This method expresses the nucleus of the lens through a smaller incision (than ICCE) at the corneal limbus by manually induced compression. The posterior lens capsule is left intact for IOL support and to keep the posterior and anterior segments apart. Though a smaller incision is created, complete visual recovery still takes 6 to 8 weeks.

- Phacoemulsification (PEM)—Phacoemulsification is the removal of the cataract through the use of an ultrasonic handpiece (versus manual expression). The nucleus is suctioned out through an opening in the titanium tip of the ultrasonic handpiece. The posterior lens capsule is left intact, as in ECCE, for support of the IOL.

PEM is performed through a 3 mm to 3.3 mm incision that is closed by a single stitch located at the corneal limbus, or is self-sealing using a clear corneal incision (also referred to as "sutureless" cataract surgery). Visual results are often apparent the next postoperative day. Complete visual recovery may vary (depending on technique) anywhere from 3 to 6 weeks.

PEM is performed within the eye as a closed system. Stability of the anterior chamber is essential for PEM to be performed safely. Large shifts in the intraocular pressure or volume of fluid in the anterior chamber during surgery will complicate the course of this procedure. Therefore, it is imperative that the surgeon and the OA be fluent in the operation of the particular type of PEM unit being used.

The preoperative parameters that the OA should note particular to PEM setup are as follows.

- The microscope is positioned with a 15° tilt of the ocular end toward the surgeon, which allows for a red reflex and enough clearance to prevent the phaco handpiece from hitting the surgeon's chest. The oculars of the microscope are set to the appropriate power and pupillary distance for the surgeon and scrub OA.

- The irrigation bottle is positioned above the cassette or pump to manufacturer's specifications; the cassette and the eye are at the same height above the floor. The bottle height is determined by the distance from the fluid level of the drip chamber to the patient's eye.

- Almost no difference in height exists between the patient's eye and the instrument tray.

- The phaco pedal is to the surgeon's left, the microscope pedal to the surgeon's right, and the wet field cautery pedal in the middle. This arrangement is best because the microscope demands finer control than the phaco pedal and is thus activated by the dominant foot.

- A neck support should be provided so the patient's head is tilted back slightly. A pillow may be placed under the patient's knees to reduce back discomfort.

- Surgical draping for the PEM method should allow easy access to the patient's airway over an appropriate drape support.

- The scrub OA should have access to the PEM machine tray, mayo stand, and back table. The circulating OA can perform important machine programming functions while doing required paperwork and be available to bring needed items into the surgical field. A video monitor facilitates awareness among the OR staff as to the particular point in the procedure.

The OA should check with the surgeon preoperatively to verify the style and power of the IOL needed for the patient. Back-up lenses should be readily available so that if the IOL to be used drops on the floor, or if complications occur requiring a change of the style, a replacement lens will be on hand.

Operative Procedure: ECCE with IOL

Prior to the procedure, the OA reassuringly stresses to the patient the importance of keeping the head still. Peribulbar or local retrobulbar anesthesia, usually consisting of marcaine 0.75% mixed with 50 units of Wydase is given in a preop holding area. Once in the OR, the OA may drape and prep the patient in the usual manner. A lid speculum is now placed in the eye and the surgery proceeds. (Figure 13-1 and 2) A fornix-based conjunctival flap is developed, exposing the surgical limbus. The OA passes the bipolar cautery to the surgeon who cauterizes the sclera and episclera.

The OA prepares a #7-0 silk traction suture on a large needleholder and hands it to the surgeon, who places it in the sclera anterior to the insertion of the superior rectus. The OA hands the ruby knife to the surgeon and a half-depth scleral groove is developed for 7 mm. A #69 blade is handed to the surgeon who develops two plane incisions into the cornea. The OA then hands a 15° blade to the surgeon who creates a paracentesis opening at 2 and 10 o'clock. The OA now passes the 6 mm spatulated sharp point blade and the surgeon creates a 3.2 mm anterior chamber incision in the pre-placed groove. A 360° capsulotomy is done using an angled 25G needle. BSS is then used to dissect the various layers of the nucleus. An atraumatic expression of the lens nucleus is performed by the surgeon. The OA prepares a #10-0 nylon suture on a fine needle holder for the surgeon to place two interrupted sutures. The OA hands the I/A handpiece to the surgeon for residual cortical removal. The posterior capsule is polished with sandblasted angled cannula. The viscoelastic agent is prepared and handed to the surgeon who places it in the posterior chamber and capsular bag. Throughout the entire procedure the OA is keeping the cornea moist for optimal visualization by the surgeon.

Both the circulator and the OA verify with the surgeon the correct IOL to open for the patient, and it is opened in the usual sterile manner. The OA hands the insertion forceps to the surgeon and the IOL is inspected for any defects. The lens is then placed into the capsular bag by the surgeon. The OA passes a Sinskey hook to the surgeon so that the lens may be rotated into position, if necessary. Then the OA hands the surgeon the bottle of BSS with an irrigation cannula tip so the remaining viscoelastic substance can be irrigated from the anterior chamber. The OA prepares acetylcholine and passes it to the surgeon. (Acetylcholine is a miotic agent that is injected intraocularly and returns the pupil to a round and regular shape). The OA at this point places a #10-0 nylon suture in a fine needleholder and passes it to the surgeon so that secure wound closure is achieved. The cautery is used to adhere the conjunctival flap. Subconjunctival injections of an antibiotic and anti-inflammatory are prepared by the OA and given to the surgeon for injection subconjunctivally. The OA patches and places a shield on the operative eye and the patient is returned to the recovery area.

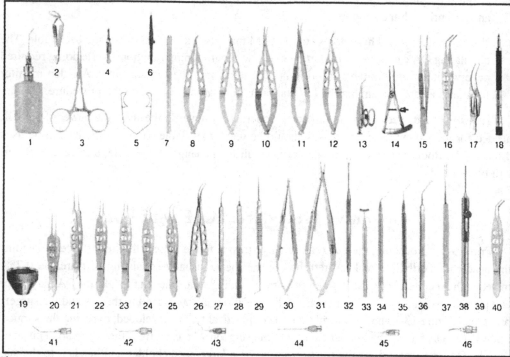

Figure 13-1. Suggested planned ECCE set. (Set illustration courtesy of Katena Products, Inc.)

1. BSS Irrigator
2. Towel Clip
3. Mosquito Forceps
4. Serrefine (2)
5. Wire Speculum
6. Super Sharp Blade
7. Blade Handle
8. Corneal Section Scissors, right
9. Corneal Section Scissors, left
10. Westcott Scissors, blunt
11. Stitch Scissors
12. Capsulotomy Scissors
13. Iris Scissors
14. Caliper
15. Conjuctiva Forceps
16. Superior Rectus Forceps
17. Colibri Forceps, 0.12 mm
18. Diamond Step Knife
19. Intraoperative Keratometer
20. Tissue Forceps
21. Suturing Forceps, 0.12 mm
22. Tying Forceps, straight
23. Tying Forceps, angled

24. Kelman-McPherson Forceps
25. Utrata Capsulorhexis Forceps
26. IOL Forceps
27. IOL Manipulator
28. Kuglen Iris Hook
29. Cyclodialysis Spatula
30. Needle Holder, micro
31. Needle Holder, standard
32. Lens Loop and Probe
33. Thornton Limbal Ruler
*34. Kansas Nucleus Trisector
*35. Kansas Nucleus Bisector
*36. Kansas Vectis, solid
*37. Kansas Nucleus Loop
*38. Keener Nucleus Divider
*39. Loop for Nucleus Divider
*40. Kansas Nucleus Fragment Forceps
41. Viscoelastic Aspirating Cannula, 22 gauge
42. Air Injection Cannula, 30 gauge
43. Viscoelastic Injection Cannula, 26 gauge
44. Cystotome
45. Capsule Polisher
46. I/A Cannula

Additional instruments for manual small incision

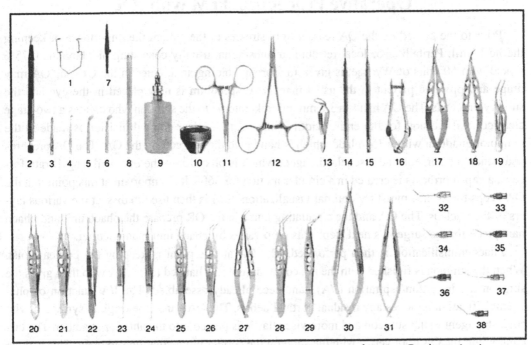

Figure 13-2. Suggested ECCE (phacoemulsification) set. (Courtesy of Katena Products, Inc.)

1. Wire Speculum
2. Diamond Knife, tri-facet
3. Keratome Blade
4. Round Blade
5. Incision Enlarging Blade, 4.0 mm
6. Incision Enlarging Blade, 5.2 mm
7. Sideport Incision Blade
8. Blade Handle (4)
9. BSS Irrigator
10. Intraoperative Keratometer
11. Mosquito Forceps, straight
12. Mosquito Forceps, curved
13. Towel Clamp
14. Nucleus Rotator
15. IOL Manipulator
16. Internal Caliper
17. Westcott Scissors, blunt
18. Capsulotomy Scissors
19. Colibri Forceps, 0.12 mm

20. Suturing Forceps, 0.12 mm
21. Superior Rectus Forceps
22. Conjuctiva Forceps
23. Tying Forceps, straight
24. Tying Forceps, curved
25. Utrata Capsulorhexis Forceps
26. Kelman-McPherson Forceps
27. IOL Forceps
*28. Soft IOL Holding Forceps
*29. Soft IOL Holding Forceps
30. Needle Holder, standard
31. Needle Holder, micro
32. Viscoelastic Aspirating Cannula, 22 gauge
33. Anterior Chamber Cannula, 30 gauge
34. Cystotome
35. Hydro-Dissection Cannula, right
36. Hydro-Dissection Cannula, left
37. Capsule Polisher
38. Viscoelastic Injection Cannula, 26 gauge

*For foldable IOLs

Operative Procedure: PEM with IOL

Prior to the procedure the OA reassuringly stresses to the patient the importance of keeping the head still. Peribulbar or local retrobulbar anesthesia, usually consisting of Marcaine 0.75% mixed with 50 units of Wydase, is given in a preop holding area. Once in the OR, the OA may drape and prep the patient in the usual manner. A speculum is now placed in the eye and the surgery proceeds. The OA hands a 3.2 mm microkeratome to the surgeon who creates a two-stage clear corneal incision for the entire width of the blade. A clear corneal incision is made in the temporal quadrant with a 15° blade which is handed to the surgeon by the OA. The OA prepares and hands the surgeon the viscoelastic agent which is placed into the eye. Utilizing Utrata forceps, a capsulorrhexis is created in a circular motion for 360°. It is important at this point that the OA keeps the cornea moist for optimal visualization. BSS is then used to dissect the various layers of the nucleus. The OA and the circulating nurse in the OR prepare the phaco unit and phaco handpiece for the surgeon's next step. This prep varies by phaco unit manufacturer.

Phacoemulsification is then performed. The OA at this point is keeping the cornea moist. When the surgeon is finished with the phaco handpiece it is handed to the OA who then gives the surgeon the irrigation/aspiration (I/A) handpiece already assembled. The I/A function of phacoemulsification removes any residual cortical debris. The OA hands the original syringe of viscoelastic agent to the surgeon and more viscoelastic is placed into the anterior chamber. The circulator and the OA both verify with the surgeon the correct intraocular lens to open. This is done in the usual sterile manner on the field. The OA then hands the insertion forceps to the surgeon and the IOL is inspected for any defects. The lens is then placed into the capsular bag by the surgeon. The OA hands the Sinskey hook to the surgeon so that the lens may be rotated into position if necessary. The OA again hands the I/A handpiece to the surgeon and any remaining viscoelastic agent is removed. The OA prepares and hands the surgeon acetylcholine, returning the pupil to a round and regular shape. Careful inspection of the corneal wound site insures non-leakage. The OA hands a collagen contact lens to the surgeon who places the lens onto the eye. (It has previously been soaked in steroid and antibiotic which had been prepared by the circulating nurse as soon as the surgery started.) The lid speculum is removed by the surgeon. A combination antibiotic/anti-inflammatory ophthalmic ointment is placed into the eye. The OA then patches and places a shield on the operative eye.

Collagen shields are used instead of subconjunctival injections for postoperative medical delivery. The shield is soaked in a combination antibiotic/corticosteroid preparation prior to placement on the operative eye. Increased patient comfort and avoidance of subconjunctival injections are a benefit realized by the use of this postoperative shield.

Complications of Cataract Surgery

Nuclear fragments dislocated into the posterior chamber are a complication of cataract surgery causing great concern to the ophthalmologist. Retained fragments of nucleus in the vitreous body may create an inflammatory response resulting in cystoid macular edema (CME), elevated IOP, and possibly corneal decompensation. In most cases, nuclear fragments are removed surgically. Conversely, small pieces of cortical material may absorb without any further complication.

The OA must be ready in the event that the surgeon asks for the vitrectomy unit should a complication arise at any time during the procedure, such as a vitreous in the anterior chamber or dislocated nuclear and cortical fragments as described above.

Gaping of a sutureless incision is another possible complication. Typically, the OA would prepare a #10-0 nylon suture on a fine needleholder for the site to be repaired by the surgeon.

Thermal burn of the sclera is a complication particular to the phacoemulsification procedure. Heat generated by the PEM tip under inadequate irrigation can cause tissues to melt rapidly at the incision site. Inadequate irrigation flow will result from bending, crimping, or disconnection of the irrigation tubing, machine pump failure, or occlusion by remaining viscoelastic material at the incision site. Careful attention to the procedure at all times by the OA will assist the surgeon in circumventing intraoperative complications.

Retina
and Vitreous

- Surgery of the retina requires fine orchestration of the various types of equipment needed simultaneously for these intraocular procedures.

- Preoperative patient instruction is important in regard to postoperative head positioning, as it is correlated to the type of procedure performed and intent of the surgery.

- Though coordination of effort between the nonsterile OR personnel and the scrub assistants is important in anticipating surgical and procedural needs in all ophthalmic procedures, surgical procedures of the retina dictate a higher level of orchestration regarding overhead room lighting, equipment changes, and multiple instrumentation at any given time.

The Retina and Vitreous Defined

The retina is a thin, transparent structure that lines the interior surface of the eye. It contains a multitude of light-sensitive nerve fibers and cells. It is often compared to the film of a camera, because the retina receives images from light that is transmitted through the optical media. These images are subsequently transmitted to the brain through the optic nerve.

The vitreous is a transparent, jelly-like substance which lies in front of the retina. It occupies most of the eye cavity.

Detachment of the posterior vitreous, or posterior vitreous detachment (PVD), may be a precursor to retinal detachment (RD). Flashing lights and floaters (cobwebs, spots) are the most commonly described symptoms of PVD. The flashing lights (photopsia) occur when the vitreous contracts and pulls on the retinal periphery.

Types of Vitreoretinal Surgery

Vitreoretinal surgery is commonly performed in the presence of RD, macular holes, diabetic retinopathy, and vitreous hemorrhage. In some cases, when tears or holes are detected before the retina actually detaches, they are sealed by means of cryotherapy (application of a cold probe to the outside of the eye wall to seal the retinal hole) or laser photocoagulation (applied directly to the retinal break). These are relatively safe and simple procedures that are usually performed on an outpatient basis.

Retinal Detachment

RD, a separation of the retina from the choroid, may be the result of tears or holes in the retinal surface. A rhegmatogenous RD is one where the tear or hole permits fluid to collect under the retina with no actual detachment. Holes or tears in the retina are often secondary to either traction (pulling) of the vitreous body because the vitreous has shrunk, or because the globe is longer than usual as in high myopia (nearsightedness). Inflammation or injury are other causes of vitreous shrinkage. Symptoms of RD include light flashes, halos around lights, loss of sectors in the field of vision, blurred vision, and many floaters. Prompt treatment of RD is necessary to prevent permanent loss of central vision. Repair of an RD is accomplished by closing the hole.

Methods of RD Repair

There are three methods that accomplish RD repair. They are scleral buckle, pneumatic retinopexy, and vitrectomy with internal gas or oil tamponade.

The scleral buckle procedure uses a circumferential or radial band to indent the sclera so that the choroid is pushed onto the retina, accomplishing closure of the hole.

In the pneumatic retinopexy procedure, expandable gas is injected into the eye, creating high surface tension, resulting in closure of the hole.

Vitrectomy is a procedure performed through the pars plana to remove vitreous gel or preretinal membranes that keep the retina detached. A gas or oil tamponade is then injected to close the hole and repair the RD.

All three techniques require sealing of the repaired hole by the use of cryo (cold probe) or application of argon/diode laser to the site.

Procedures for Diabetic Retinopathy (DR)

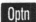

Diabetic retinopathy is a direct complication of diabetes, resulting in leakage from blood vessels within the retinal tissue. Neovascularization (abnormal growth of fragile, aberrant vessels) also occurs, causing leakage and scarring. Leakage of blood may also occur directly into the vitreous gel creating a vitreous hemorrhage. For the patient, the result of any of these conditions is decreased vision.

The longer a person has diabetes, the higher the risk of developing DR. About 80% of those who have had diabetes for at least 15 years have some blood vessel damage to the retina. People with Type I (juvenile) diabetes are more likely to develop DR at a younger age.

DR is classified as either background (BDR), an early stage of leakage with resultant edema, or proliferative (PDR), when new, abnormal blood vessels begin growing on the surface of the retina.

Panretinal photocoagulation (PRP) laser surgery has been shown to reduce the risk of severe vision loss from PDR.

Operative Procedure: Scleral Buckle Procedure for Rhegmatogenous RD Utilizing Intravitreal Gas

Prior to the start of the procedure, the scrub OA (after appropriate sterile gowning and gloving) drapes the mayo stand in sterile technique. In conjunction with the nonsterile circulating OA, the surgical microscope is draped according to sterile technique with eyepieces exposed so that sterile eyepiece covers can be applied. The instrument tray is organized, suture materials prepared, and cryo equipment verified to be operational. (Figure 14-1)

Either general anesthesia or local with anesthesia stand-by is administered to the patient upon arrival in the OR. The patient is placed in the supine position, the operative eye (as identified by either the OA or the attending surgeon) is prepped and draped according to sterile protocol.

A lid speculum is inserted by the attending surgeon. A 360° peritomy is performed using Westcott scissors. The conjunctiva is bluntly dissected with Tenon's conjunctival scissors. The OA prepares a #4-0 silk on a needleholder. The rectus muscles are isolated and the muscle hooked with #4-0 silk sutures. The sclera is inspected for thinning. The circulating OA places the nonsterile indirect ophthalmoscope on the surgeon's head and adjusts it appropriately. The scrub OA passes the sterile 20 diopter indirect lens to the surgeon. Using this lens, indirect ophthalmoscopy is performed and the retinal detachment is located. Inspection of the retina is made to identify all holes or tears. All of the tears are marked with a diathermy (heat coagulation) marking pencil. The OA hands the sterile cryo probe to the surgeon and cryotherapy is applied. The surgeon decides at this point to place either a circumferential or radial buckle. (For example, if the decision is to place a circumferential buckle and the tear is at 6 o'clock, the surgeon will place a horizontal mattress suture in the inferotemporal and inferonasal quadrant.) The width of suture placement is in direct correlation to the type and size of buckling material chosen. (For example, a 7 mm sponge would require a horizontal mattress suture, placed 9.5 mm to 10 mm apart.)

After the buckle is placed, and before the sutures are tied over the buckling material, the subretinal fluid is drained via a scleral incision made with a #57 blade down through the choroid until the subretinal space is penetrated. A #5-0 nylon suture is prepared on a locking needleholder and passed to the surgeon. Buckling material, either band or sponge, is passed to the attending surgeon by the OA, and it is placed for 360° around the globe.

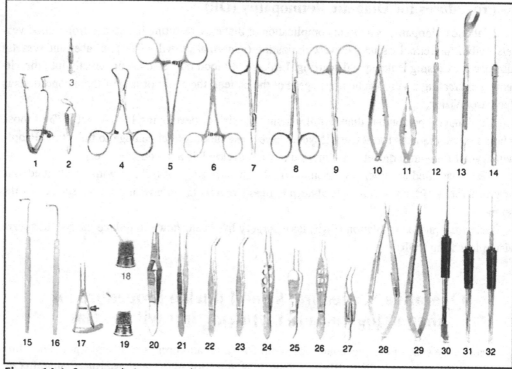

Figure 14-1. *Suggested vitreo-retinal set. (Set illustration courtesy of Katena Products, Inc.)*

1. Eye Speculum, large
2. Baby Towel Clamp 2 1/4" (2)
3. Serrefine (4)
4. Towel Clamp 3 1/2" (2)
5. Mosquito Forceps (2)
6. Baby Mosquito Forceps (2)
7. Eye Scissors, straight
8. Eye Scissors, curved
9. Stevens Scissors
10. Westcott Scissors, right
11. Vannas Scissors
12. Blade Handle (2), K-Blade #64
13. Orbital Retractor
14. Stiletto Blade (20 gauge) and handle
15. Muscle Hook, large
16. Retinal Detachment Hook (2)

17. Caliper
18. Scleral Marker
19. Scleral Depressor
20. Sleeve Spreading Forceps
21. Conjuctiva Forceps 1.2 mm (2)
22. Utility Forceps, smooth
23. Utility Forceps, serrated
24. Suturing Forceps 0.12 mm
25. Fixation Forceps 1x2
26. Tying Forceps, straight (2)
27. Colibri Forceps 0.12 mm
28. Needle Holder, straight
29. Needle Holder, curved
30. Intraocular Scissors, angled
31. Intraocular Fordeps, serrated
32. Intraocular Forceps with platform

Following the drainage, the OA prepares the #6-0 Vicryl suture on a nonlocking needleholder. The sclerotomy site is closed with a #6-0 Vicryl suture. The wound site is inspected closely by the surgeon for any evidence of hemorrhage or incarceration at the drain site. At this point, the horizontal mattress suture is tied over the buckle. To see if the hole is closed over the buckle, indirect ophthalmoscopy is performed. If the hole is not totally closed over the buckle, injection of pure intravitreal sulfahexafluoride (SF-6) gas would be indicated. The amount of SF-6 gas injected is appropriately noted by the surgeon to the circulating OA (usually .25 cc to .33 cc). This gas expands slightly to keep the hole closed against the buckle. If the intraocular pressure is increased, a paracentesis is performed with a #30 gauge needle on a tuberculosis (TB) syringe to bring the pressure down. The #4-0 silk rectus sutures are then removed, and the conjunctiva is closed with a #6-0 plain or #8-0 Vicryl suture. Dexamethasone ointment, patch, and shield are applied to the eye by the OA. If gas has been injected, it is necessary for the OA to explain to the patient the importance of postoperative head positioning. The bubble must always be above the repaired site, as it pushes against the tear. Opposite head positioning would negate the goal of the procedure.

Silicone oil is another type of vitreous substitute. This material is used for treating severe, complicated RDs. It is a clear, synthetic liquid that creates an internal tamponade by pushing the retina against the inside back wall of the eye. It is often surgically removed after 3 to 4 months. Silicone oil is primarily used in eyes that have had previous surgery for RD.

Procedure: Pars Plana Vitrectomy with Membrane Peel

A membrane peel would be indicated in cases of macular pucker, severe proliferative vitreo-retinopathy (PVR), and RD.

Prior to the start of the procedure, the scrub OA (after appropriate sterile gowning and gloving) drapes the mayo stand in sterile fashion. In conjunction with the nonsterile circulating OA, the surgical microscope is draped in sterile fashion with eyepieces exposed so that sterile eyepiece covers can be applied. The instrument tray is organized, and general or local anesthesia with standby is established. Vitrectomy and laser equipment are verified to be operational.

After the patient is placed in the supine position, the operative eye is identified by either the OA or the attending surgeon. The patient is then draped in appropriate sterile fashion by the OA. A lid speculum is placed on the operative eye by the surgeon.

The OA passes Westcott scissors to the attending surgeon. Incisions are made superotemporally, superonasally, and inferotemporally into the conjunctiva and Tenon's capsule. Hemostasis is maintained by the attending surgeon, utilizing a wet field bipolar cautery. During this maneuver, the OA is responsible for keeping the operative site dry utilizing a cotton-tipped applicator. A caliper is passed to the surgeon who measures 3.5 mm to 4 mm from the limbus to determine the entry site of the ora serrata (the junction of the peripheral retina and ciliary body) to avoid causing an RD. This site is marked with the tips of the caliper. A #5-0 nylon suture is prepared by the OA and passed to the surgeon, who places it in the inferotemporal area centered 3.5 mm to 4 mm posterior to the limbus. This suture will eventually hold the infusion cannula.

The OA passes an microvitreoretinal (MVR) knife to the surgeon and a sclerostomy is made at the site. An #8-0 Vicryl suture is prepared by the OA on a locking needleholder and passed to the surgeon. The suture is placed over the sclerotomy site. An infusion cannula for BSS infusion is placed at the sclerotomy site by the surgeon and tied down with the pre-placed #5-0 nylon suture. The surgeon then inspects the area to insure the infusion cannula is well within the vitreous cavity so that the fluid will always flow into the vitreous cavity. The surgeon observes the depth of the vitreous cavity through the microscope, usually with an irrigation contact lens. The space between the cornea and contact lens must not contain air because the cornea may dry out, making visibility difficult.

The OA passes the MVR knife to the surgeon for sclerostomies to be made superotemporally and superonasally centered 3.5 mm to 4 mm posterior to the limbus. The OA connects the light pipe from the vitrectomy unit (which will illuminate the interior of the globe) and passes it to the surgeon. After the core vitrectomy is performed with a side-cutting instrument, the surgeon inspects for any areas of vitreoretinal traction or preretinal fibrosis that may extend from the optic disc to the macular area. If found to be significant, the traction (pulling) is released by a membrane peel technique. The OA passes the 20 diopter lens to the surgeon and indirect ophthalmoscopy is again performed to inspect for any further breaks or tears in the retina.

The OA then prepares a #8-0 Vicryl on a needleholder and passes the suture to the surgeon, who closes the sclerostomies. The previously-placed infusion cannula is then removed and the site closed with the pre-placed #8-0 Vicryl suture. The conjunctiva and Tenon's capsule are closed using the #8-0 Vicryl suture. The OA draws injections of betamethasone sodium phosphate {Celestone (Schering Corp., Kenilworth, NJ)} and cefazolin for sub-Tenon injection by the surgeon. The OA applies an antibiotic ointment and then patches and shields the operative eye.

General Assisting Notes

- Attention to the level of room lighting throughout retinal procedures is essential in providing the surgeon and OR team adequate visualization during surgery.

- Standard BSS bottle height is kept at 2 feet above the eye. However, the surgeon may have the scrub OA adjust the bottle height to control intraocular conditions. (For example, the bottle height would be raised to control intraocular bleeding.)

- To avoid accidental tripping, circulating personnel in the OR must be aware of equipment cord placement on the floor surrounding the surgeon. This is especially important in retinovitreous procedures where the room may be dark for most of the case.

- A system of effective management and disposal of irrigation solutions must be in place at the start of the surgery to prevent fluid from soaking the surgeon and patient. This is usually accomplished by creating a collection "moat" from the ends of the eye drape around the patient's head. It is also important to protect equipment pedals with plastic covers to prevent fluid from shorting out the electrical components.

- Finally, all patients who undergo vitreoretinal surgery must be instructed to contact their ophthalmologist immediately if they experience any loss of vision, flashes of light, or new floaters.

Bibliography

Alpar JJ. *Ophthalmic Surgery.* New York, NY: Raven Press Books Ltd; 1987.

Boyd-Monk H, Steinmetz CG. *Operating Room Procedures: Nursing Care of the Eye.* Norwalk, CT: Appleton & Lange; 1987.

Brandt J. Glaucoma. *LEO Clinical Topic Update.* San Francisco, CA: American Academy of Ophthalmology; 1995.

Care and Handling of Diamond Knives. METICO Instrument Division of AKORN Inc. Abita Springs, LA.

Cassin B, ed. *Fundamentals for Ophthalmic Technical Personnel.* Philadelphia, PA: WB Saunders Company; 1995.

Cassin B, Solomon S. *Dictionary of Eye Terminology.* Gainesville, FL: Triad Publishing Company; 1990.

Charters L. Conjunctival miniautograft may end pterygium recurrences. *Ophthalmology Times.* 1996; 21(4):39-41.

Corneal Diseases and Surgery. [public education pamphlet]. Philadelphia, PA: Wills Eye Hospital; 1994.

Detached And Torn Retina. [public education pamphlet]. San Francisco, CA: American Academy of Ophthalmology; 1992.

Diabetic Retinopathy. [public education pamphlet]. San Francisco, CA: American Academy of Ophthalmology; 1995.

Don't Lose Sight of Diabetic Eye Disease: Information for People with Diabetes. [public education pamphlet]. National Eye Health Education Program. National Eye Institute: Bethesda, MD; Publication No 93-3252.

External Disease and Cornea. Basic Clinical and Science Course. San Francisco, CA: American Academy of Ophthalmology; 1990.

Eye Facts About: Corneal Disease and Transplants. [public education pamphlet]. San Francisco, CA: American Academy of Ophthalmology; 1986.

Eye Facts About: Keratoconus. [public education pamphlet]. San Francisco, CA: American Academy of Ophthalmology; 1987.

Eye Facts About: Pterygium and Pingueculum. [public education pamphlet]. San Francisco, CA: American Academy of Ophthalmology; 1988.

Glaucoma. [public education pamphlet]. San Francisco, CA: American Academy of Ophthalmology; 1993.

Guidelines for Caring for Micro Instruments. METICO Instrument Division of AKORN Inc. Abita Springs, LA.

Instrument Care Book. Denville, NJ: Katena Products, Inc; 1991.

Jackson-Williams B. *Ophthalmic Surgical Assisting.* 2nd ed. Thorofare, NJ: SLACK Inc.; 1993.

Kronemyer B. Pterygium: Conjunctival autograft tailor-made for developing countries. *Ocular Surgery News.* 1996; 14(15):39-41.

LASIK—A New Horizon in Laser Vision Correction. [public education pamphlet]. Houston, TX: Patient Education Concepts, Inc.; 1997.

Lavrich JB, Nelson LB. Diagnosis and Treatment of Strabismus Disorders. *Pediatric Ophthalmology.* 1993; 40(4):737-752.

Machat JJ. *Excimer Laser Refractive Surgery—Practices and Principles.* Thorofare, NJ: SLACK Inc; 1996.

Meeker MH, Rothrock JC. *Alexander's Care of the Patient in Surgery.* 10th ed. St. Louis, MO: Mosby-Year Book Inc; 1995.

Melton R, Thomas R. The 1996 Clinical Guide to Ophthalmic Drugs. Supplement to *Review of Optometry.* 1996; 133(5):17A.

Minckler DS, Shammas A, Wilcox M, et al. Experimental studies of aqueous filtration using the Molteno implant. *Trans American Ophthalmological Society.* 1987; 85:368-392.

Nelson LB, Lavrich JB, eds. *Strabismus Surgery—Ophthalmology Clinics of North America.* Philadelphia, PA: WB Saunders Company; 1992: 5(1).

Nordan LT, Maxwell WA, Davison JA, eds. *The Surgical Rehabilitation of Vision.* New York, NY: Gower Medical Publishing; 1992.

Pediatric Ophthalmology. [public education pamphlet]. Philadelphia, PA: Wills Eye Hospital; 1995.

Precursors of Rhegmatogenous Retinal Detachment in Adults. Preferred Practice Pattern. San Francisco, CA: The American Academy of Ophthalmology; 1994.

Proposed Recommended Practices—Sterilization. Denver, CO: *AORN Journal*; 1991; 54(1):82-94.

Proposed Recommended Practices for Sterilization in the Practice Setting. Denver, CO: *AORN Journal*; 1994; 60(1):109-119.

Recommended Practices—Disinfection. Denver, CO: *AORN Journal.* 1992; 56(4):715-719.

Recommended Practices—Steam and Ethylene Oxide (EO) Sterilization. Denver, CO: *AORN Journal*;1992; 56(4):721-730.

Repka MX. Pediatric ophthalmology and strabismus. *LEO Clinical Topic Update.* San Francisco, CA: American Academy of Ophthalmology; 1996.

Report of the American Society of Cataract and Refractive Surgery International Committee on Standards and Quality Control for Ophthalmic Instruments and Devices. *Journal of Cataract and Refractive Surgery;* 1991; 17:359-365.

Retinal Detachment. Preferred Practice Pattern. San Francisco, CA: The American Academy of Ophthalmology; 1990.

Retinal Detachment Surgery and Vitrectomy. [public education pamphlet]. Philadelphia, PA: Wills Eye Hospital; 1993.

Rhode SJ, Ginsberg SP. *Ophthalmic Technology—A Guide for the Eye Care Assistant.* New York, NY: Raven Press; 1987.

Rubin SE, Nelson LB. *Complications of Strabismus Surgery—Ophthalmology Clinics of North America.* Philadelphia, PA: WB Saunders Company; 1992; 5(1): 157-163.

Sigelman J. *Retinal Diseases - Pathogenesis, Laser Therapy, and Surgery.* 1st ed. Boston, MA: Little, Brown and Company; 1984.

Smith JF, Nachazel DP. *Ophthalmologic Nursing.* 1st ed. Boston, MA: Little, Brown, and Company; 1980.

Spalton DJ, Hitchings RA, Hunter PA. *Atlas of Clinical Ophthalmology.* New York, NY: Gower Medical Publishing; 1984.

Standards and Recommended Practices. Denver, CO: Association of Operating Room Nurses, Inc; 1996.

Stein HA, Slatt BJ, Stein RA. *The Ophthalmic Assistant—Fundamentals and Clinical Practice.* 5th ed. St. Louis, MO: CV Mosby Co; 1988.

Stein HA, Slatt BJ, Stein RA. *The Ophthalmic Assistant—Fundamentals and Clinical Practice.* 6th ed. St. Louis, MO: CV Mosby Co; 1994.

Stein HA, Slatt BJ, Stein RA. *Ophthalmic Terminology.* 3rd ed. St Louis, MO: Mosby- Year Book, Inc.; 1993.

Surgery of the Extraocular Muscles. Basic Clinical and Science Course. San Francisco, CA: American Academy of Ophthalmology; 1990.

Suture Materials. *Physician's Desk Reference for Ophthalmology.* 25th ed. Montvale NJ; 1997.

Tipperman R, Lichtenstein SB. Cataract. Advances in Clinical Diagnosis—Measurement of Visual Function. *LEO Clinical Topic Update.* San Francisco, CA: American Academy of Ophthalmology; 1996.

Tipperman R, Lichtenstein SB. Cataract. Anesthesia. *LEO Clinical Topic Update.* San Francisco, CA: American Academy of Ophthalmology; 1996.

Understanding Laser Vision Correction. [public education pamphlet]. Rockville, MD: TLC 20/20 Laser Services; 1998.

Understanding PRK—Techniques and Technology. Supplement to *Review of Ophthalmology.* 1996; 3(5).

Use and Care of Titanium Surgical Instruments. Solan Ophthalmic Products. Jacksonville, FL.

Waltman SR, Krupin T. *Complications in Ophthalmic Surgery.* Philadelphia, PA: JB Lippincott Company; 1980.

Yang-Williams K. Optometric and Medical Abbreviations. *Review of Optometry.* 1997; 134(2):121-124.

Zabel K. Anterior chamber lidocaine aids in surgery. *Ophthalmology Times;* 1997; 22(5):21.

Appendix

Abbreviations
and Acronyms

Abbreviations and Acronyms

3D	3 Dimensional
5-FU	5-Fluorouracil (antimetabolite)
AACG	Acute Angle Closure Glaucoma
a.c.	Before Meals
AC	Anterior Chamber
ACD	Anterior Chamber Depth
ACG	Angle Closure Glaucoma
ACL	Anterior Chamber Lens
ACM	Anterior Chamber Maintainer
AFGE	Air Fluid Gas Exchange
AIDS	acquired immunodeficiency syndrome
AL	Axial Length
ALT	Argon Laser Trabeculoplasty
amp.	Ampule
AORN	Association of Operating Room Nurses, Inc.
ARMD	Age Related Macular Degeneration
ASA	Aspirin (acetylsalicylic acid)
ASAP	As Soon As Possible
ASC	Ambulatory Surgery Center
ASC	Anterior Subcapsular Cataract
ASCVD	Atherosclerotic Cardiovascular Disease
Avx	Anterior Vitrectomy
BAO	Branch Artery Occlusion
BAT	Brightness Acuity Testing
BCC	Basal Cell Carcinoma
BDR	Background Diabetic Retinopathy
b.i.d.	Twice a Day
BP	Blood Pressure
BRAO	Branch Retinal Artery Occlusion
BRVO	Branch Retinal Vein Occlusion
BS	Blind Spot
BSS	Balanced Salt Solution
BVA	Best Visual Acuity
Bx	Biopsy
C & S	Culture & Sensitivity
CA	Carcinoma
CA	Corneal Abrasion
CAD	Coronary Artery Disease
CBC	Complete Blood Count
cc	Cubic Centimeter
c.c.	Latin for *cum correctio* (With Correction)

CC	Chief Complaint
C/D	Cup-to-Disc Ratio
CE	Cataract Extraction
CHF	Congestive Heart Failure
CME	Cystoid Macular Edema
CMV	Cytomegalovirus
cm	Centimeter
CN	Cranial Nerve
CNS	Central Nervous System
c/o	Complains Of
COAG	Chronic Open Angle Glaucoma
COLD	Chronic Obstructive Lung Disease
conj	Conjunctiva
COPD	Chronic Obstructive Pulmonary Disease
CPC	Cyclophotocoagulation (laser)
CPK	Creatinine Phosphokinase enzyme
CRA	Central Retinal Artery
CRAO	Central Retinal Artery Occlusion
CRV	Central Retinal Vein
CRVO	Central Retinal Vein Occlusion
CSM	Central, Steady, and Maintained (Fixation)
CSR	Central Serous Retinopathy
CT	Computerized Axial Tomography or CAT Scan
CVA	Cerebrovascular Accident (Stroke)
CVD	Cardiovascular Disease
cyl	Cylinder
D	Diopter
DCR	Dacryocystorhinostomy
DD	Disc Diameter (Optic)
DM	Diabetes Mellitus
DMV	Disc, Macula, Vessels
DR	Diabetic Retinopathy
DVM	Disc, Vessels, Macula
Dx	Diagnosis
ECC	Endothelial Cell Count
ECCE	Extracapsular Cataract Extraction
ECG	Electrocardiogram
e.g	Latin for *exempli gratia* (For Example)
EKG	Electrocardiogram
EO	Ethylene Oxide
EOM	Extraocular Muscle(s)
EOMB	Extraocular Muscle Balance
ERG	Electroretinography
ERM	Epiretinal Membrane

ETOH	Ethanol; alcohol (used in reference to alcohol abuse)
EUA	Examination Under Anesthesia
FA	Fluorescein Angiogram (or Angiography)
FB	Foreign Body
FBS	Foreign Body Sensation
FH	Family History
f/u	Follow-up
Fx	Fracture
GPC	Giant Papillary Conjunctivitis
GTT	Glucose Tolerance Test
gtts	Latin for *guttae* (Drops)
Hb	Hemoglobin
HBP	High Blood Pressure
Hct	Hematocrit
HCTZ	Hydrochlorthiazide
HCVD	Hypertensive Cardiovascular Disease
Hgb	Hemoglobin
HIV	human immunodeficiency virus
Hg	Mercury
HK	Herpes Keratitis
HM	Hand Motion (or movement) Vision
H+P	History and Physical
HPI	History of Present Illness
HR	Heart Rate
h.s.	At Bedtime/Hour of Sleep
HS	Herpes Simplex
HSK	Herpes Simplex Keratitis
HSV	Herpes Simplex Virus
HTN	Hypertension
Hx	History
I/A	Irrigation/Aspiration
i.c.	Between Meals
ICCE	Intracapsular Cataract Extraction
ICU	Intensive Care Unit
I & D	Incision & Drainage
IDDM	Insulin-Dependent Diabetes Mellitus
i.e.	Latin for *id est* (That is)
IgA	Immunoglobulin A
IgD	Immunoglobulin D
IgE	Immunoglobulin E (hypersensitivity reactions)
IgG	Immunoglobulin G (bacterial and viral infections)
IgM	Immunoglobulin M (bacterial and viral infections)

IHD	Ischemic Heart Disease
IK	Interstitial Keratitis
IM	Intramuscularly
IO	Inferior Oblique (muscle)
IOFB	Intraocular Foreign Body
IOL	Intraocular Lens
ION	Ischemic Optic Neuropathy
IOP	Intraocular Pressure
IV	Intravenous or Intravitreal
IVFA	Intravenous Fluorescein Angiography
J	Jaeger Visual Acuity
K	Keratometry
K	Potassium
KS	Keratitis Sicca
K sicca	Keratoconjunctivitis sicca
LASER	Light Amplification by Stimulated Emission of Radiation
LASIK	Laser in situ Keratomileusis
LE	Lupus Erythematosus
LI	Laser Interferometry
LK	Lamellar Keratoplasty
LL	Lower Lid
LP	Light Perception
LPI	Laser Peripheral Iridotomy
LR	Lateral Rectus (muscle)
LTG	Low Tension Glaucoma
LTK	Laser Thermokeratoplasty
LTP	Laser Trabeculoplasty
m	Meter
MAC	Monitored Anesthesia Care
mg	Milligram
MG	Myasthenia Gravis or Marcus Gunn (pupil)
MH	Malignant Hyperthermia
MKM	Myopic Keratomileusis
ml	Milliliter
mm	Millimeter
MR	Medial Rectus (muscle)
MRI	Magnetic Resonance Imaging
MS	Multiple Sclerosis
N & V	Nausea & Vomiting
NA	Not Applicable
NCQA	National Committee on Quality Assurance

Nd:YAG	Neodymium: Yttrium-Aluminum-Garnet (laser)
neo	Neovascularization
Neo	Neosynephrine
NFL	Nerve Fiber Layer
NKA	No Known Drug Allergies
NLD	Nasolacrimal Duct
NLP	No Light Perception
NPA	Near Point of Accommodation
NPC	Near Point of Convergence
NPO	Nothing by Mouth
NS	Nuclear Sclerosis or Non Smoker
NSAID	Non-steroidal Anti-inflammatory Drug
NVD	Neovascularization of the Disc
NVE	Neovascularization Elsewhere
NVG	Neovascular Glaucoma
OD	Latin for *oculus dexter* (Right Eye)
ODM	Ophthalmodynamometry
OHT	Ocular Hypertension
OMP	Ophthalmic Medical Personnel
ON	Optic Nerve
ONH	Optic Nerve Head
ONSD	Optic Nerve Sheath Decompression
OR	Operating Room
OS	Latin for *oculus sinistra* (Left Eye)
OSHA	Occupational Safety and Health Administration
OTC	Over The Counter
OU	Latin for *oculus uterque* (Both Eyes)
OZ	Optical Zone
P & I	Probing & Irrigation (Lacrimal System)
PAM	Potential Acuity Meter
PAS	Peripheral Anterior Synechia
p.c.	After Meals
PC	Posterior Capsule or Posterior Chamber
PCL	Posterior Chamber Lens
PCN	Pencillin
PDR	Physicians Desk Reference
PDR	Proliferative Diabetic Retinopathy
PE	(Retinal) Pigment Epithelium
PEM	Phacoemulsification
PERRLA	Pupils Equal, Round, and Reactive to Light and Accommodation
PH	Past History
PH	Pinhole Visual Acuity
PHNI	Pinhole No Improvement
PI	Peripheral Iridectomy (or Iridotomy)

PKP	Penetrating Keratoplasty
PMH	Past Medical History
PMMA	Polymethyl Methacrylate
PNS	Peripheral Nervous System
PO	Latin *per os* (by mouth)
po	Postoperative
PP	Punctal Plug or Pressure Patch
PP	Pars Plana
PPDR	Preproliferative Diabetic Retinopathy
PPL	Pars Plana Lensectomy
PPV	Pars Plana Vitrectomy
PRH	Preretinal Hemorrhage
PRK	Photorefractive Keratectomy
p.r.n.	Latin for *pro re nata* (as needed)
PRP	Pan Retinal Photocoagulation
PRRE	Pupils Round, Regular & Equal
PSC	Posterior Subcapsular Cataract
PTK	Phototherapeutic Keratectomy
PTP	Part Time Patch
PVD	Posterior Vitreous Detachment
PVR	Proliferative Vitreoretinopathy
P$_x$	Prognosis
q.d.	Every Day
q.h.	Every Hour
q.h.s.	Every Bedtime
q.i.d.	Four Times a Day
q.o.d.	Every Other Day
q3h	Every 3 Hours
RA	Rheumatoid Arthritis
RB	Retinoblastoma
RBC	Red Blood Cell
RD	Retinal Detachment
Ref	Refraction
RH	Retinal Hemorrhage
RK	Radial Keratotomy
RLF	Retrolental Fibroplasia
RLR	Right Lateral Rectus (muscle)
RN	Registered Nurse
r/o	Rule Out
ROP	Retinopathy of Prematurity
ROS	Review of Systems
RP	Retinitis Pigmentosa
RPE	Retinal Pigment Epithelium
RPED	Retinal Pigment Epithelium Detachment
Rx	Prescribed Treatment

s	Without
S	Sphere
SB	Scleral Buckling Procedure
sc	Subcutaneous
s.c.	Without Correction
SCH	Subconjunctival Hemorrhage
SCH	Suprachoroidal Hemorrhage
SF	Sulfa Hexafluoride
SFG	Sulfa Hexafluoroide Gas
SLE	Slit Lamp Exam
SLE	Systemic Lupus Erythematosus
SMCD	Senile Macular and Choroidal Degeneration
SMD	Senile Macular Degeneration
SOV	Superior Ophthalmic Vein
SRF	Subretinal Fluid
SRH	Subretinal Hemorrhage
SRM	Subretinal Membrane
SRN	Subretinal Neovascularization
SRNV	Subretinal Neovascularization
SRNVM	Subretinal Neovascular Membrane
stat	Immediately
STT	Schirmer Tear Testing
subcut.	Subcutaneous (under the skin)
sub q	Subcutaneous (under the skin)
Sx	Symptom
SX	Surgery
TB	Tuberculosis (as in TB syringe)
TBUT	Tear Break Up Time
TIA	Transient Ischemic Attack
t.i.d.	Three Times a Day
TM	Trabecular Meshwork
TNF	Tension Normal by Finger (palpation)
TNTC	Too Numerous to Count
TPPL	Trans Pars Plana Lensectomy
TPPV	Trans Pars Plana Vitrectomy
TRD	Total Retinal Detachment
TRD	Traction Retinal Detachment
Tx	Treatment
UGH	Uveitis, Glaucoma, Hyphema
UL	Upper Lid
ung	Ointment
US	Ultrasound
UV	Ultraviolet

VA	Visual Acuity
VDRL	Venereal Disease Research Laboratory
VEP	Visual Evoked Potential
VER	Visual Evoked Response
VF	Visual Field
Vit.	Vitreous
VS	Vital Signs
V/S	Vital Signs
WNL	Within Normal Limits
w/u	Work-up
YAG	Yttrium-Aluminum-Garnet (laser)
y/o	Years Old

Index

Printed in the United States
by Baker & Taylor Publisher Services